# Emotion and Healing
## in the
# Energy Body

"What lays between your 'true' and 'current' self? Based on Robert Henderson's thorough, enriching, and illuminating explanations of subtle energy and healing, I would say, 'Your place of power.' Henderson's brilliant book outlines the means for detecting the blocked energies in your life and body and ways to clear them using energetic, yogic, and massage processes. Henderson's comprehensive understanding of the sources of our obvious problems, from karma to emotions to mental misunderstandings, will enable us all to powerfully transform others and ourselves."

CYNDI DALE, AUTHOR OF
*THE SUBTLE BODY, NEW CHAKRA HEALING,*
*ENERGETIC BOUNDARIES,* AND *THE INTUITION GUIDEBOOK*

"With more than 15 years of experience teaching and practicing Thai massage, Robert's book enriches the culture of massage and yoga. In clear and simple language he provides a doorway to understanding the role of energy in healing. I highly recommend this book for those who want to explore beyond the physical."

KAM THYE CHOW, FOUNDER AND DIRECTOR OF
THE LOTUS PALM SCHOOL AND AUTHOR OF
*THAI YOGA MASSAGE* AND
*THAI YOGA THERAPY FOR YOUR BODY TYPE*

# Emotion and Healing
## in the
# Energy Body

### A HANDBOOK OF
### SUBTLE ENERGIES
### IN MASSAGE AND YOGA

## ROBERT HENDERSON

Healing Arts Press
Rochester, Vermont • Toronto, Canada

Healing Arts Press
One Park Street
Rochester, Vermont 05767
www.HealingArtsPress.com

Healing Arts Press is a division of Inner Traditions International

*Note to the reader: This book is intended as an informational guide. The remedies, approaches, and techniques described herein are meant to supplement, and not to be a substitute for, professional medical care or treatment. They should not be used to treat a serious ailment without prior consultation with a qualified health care professional.*

**Library of Congress Cataloging-in-Publication Data**
Henderson, Robert, 1962– , author.
  Emotion and healing in the energy body : a handbook of subtle energies in massage and yoga / Robert Henderson.
      p. ; cm.
  Includes index.
  Summary: "A comprehensive guide to emotional blockages in the energy body and their physical manifestations"—Provided by publisher.
  ISBN 978-1-62055-427-2 (pbk.) — ISBN 978-1-62055-428-9 (e-book)
  I. Title.
  [DNLM: 1.  Mental Healing. 2.  Emotions—physiology. 3.  Massage. 4.  Qi. 5. Yoga.  WB 880]
  RZ421
  615.8'52—dc23
                                                                    2014045693

Printed and bound in the United States by Versa Press, Inc.

10  9  8  7  6  5  4  3  2  1

Text design by Priscilla H. Baker and layout by Virginia Scott Bowman
This book was typeset in Garamond Premier Pro and Gill Sans with Sabon and Fruitger used as display typefaces

To send correspondence to the author of this book, mail a first-class letter to the author c/o Inner Traditions • Bear & Company, One Park Street, Rochester, VT 05767, and we will forward the communication, or contact the author directly at **www.roberthenderson.info**.

*I dedicate this book to my spiritual family:*
*Mary Kavanagh, my mother, Brian Henderson,*
*my father, and John G. Kavanagh, my grandfather.*
*And to my grandmother, Anna O'Keeffe,*
*who in spirit oversaw everything.*

# Contents

# Acknowledgments

This book marks the end of a fifteen-year phase in my life. Looking back it is easy to trace the linear, sequential line of people who came into my life, guiding me, like geography guides a river, to my current destination. Although there are too many people to thank individually, there are some people I want to give deserved recognition to.

Thank you . . .

Shaun Cotter, my old flatmate in London who first introduced me to yoga.

My Thai massage teachers: Asokananda, who showed me how to do it, and Chaiyuth Priyasith, who showed me what you can do with it.

Jasmine Vishnu, my energy teacher in Chiang Mai.

Radha and Pierre at Yoga Plus in Crete, where, working as a massage therapist, I was able to bridge the elements of Thai massage and energy work.

Max Scheuermeier at the Sunshine Massage School in Chiang Mai where I developed and taught my first courses on energy work in Thai massage.

Jon Graham and Meghan MacLean at Inner Traditions for their support and guidance in publishing this book. As learning leads to practice, so practice leads to teaching and teaching leads to writing.

Finally, to Vienna and to Elfi Mayr of Yogaguide who helped me find my feet.

And very finally, a big thank you to Nathalie Mayer, *Supergirl*.

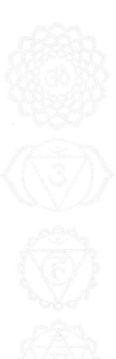

PART ONE

# Introduction to Subtle Energy and the Chakras

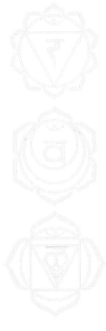

# 1

# Understanding Subtle Energy

It can be difficult to explain what subtle energy is to someone who has never had any direct experience of it. It's like trying to describe electricity—you know it exists, and you have a good idea of what it does, but you have no real concept of what it is experientially until you touch a live wire and feel the effects surging through your body. Then you begin to truly understand what electricity is and can even find words to describe it. It is the same with energy. You have to touch it, you have to experience it and feel its effects, before you can understand what it is.

When you first begin to tune in to the subtle energy of your body, you discover that there are different types of energy, such as the energy that powers the mental determination to get something done, or the emotional energy that gives rise to feelings of sadness or joy. Upon closer examination of emotional energy, you will discover that each emotion has its own unique feel, its own unique energy stamp, and that each one is unique and different from the others. For example, the emotional energy of loneliness feels quite different from the emotional energy of anger, and they affect your body in different ways, too. The energy of anger makes muscles become agitated and hard, creating reduced flexibility and mobility and increased resistance, or physical discomfort, when you move them, whereas the emotional energy of loneliness manifests as deep coldness, causing muscles to contract and tighten. In time you will discover how all the different emotions feel in your body, where you store them in your body, and the specific effect each one has on your body—a subject we'll be exploring in greater detail in the coming chapters.

By examining the body's subtle energies, you will come to understand that many of the physical discomforts experienced in the body are caused by some form of subtle-energy blockage. Knowing this, of course, can help you discover an appropriate course of action to take to help alleviate any discomfort or pain you may be experiencing. For instance, if you have a sexual partner who is transmitting unhealthy sexual energy into you, you will experience this as a feeling of weakness in your lower back and a low-level, constant nausea. Upon feeling this, you may go to the drugstore or to the doctor for help, but the root cause of what is really making you sick is the sexual energy you have been taking in from your partner. Remove the source of the discomfort and the discomfort will go away. This principle is fundamental to true healing. Going to the doctor, in this example, would only be papering over the cracks.

This is why understanding what subtle energy is can be such a help in understanding what makes your body the way it is, what makes you feel the way you do, and what makes you do the things you do. The understanding of subtle-body energy becomes a whole new way of connecting to yourself, reading your body, communicating with it, and understanding what it is telling you about your life. In the end it shows you that your body is your best guide to telling you everything you need to know about your life—where you have been, where you are going, and, most importantly, the things you need to do to stay on the path that will bring you the greatest rewards and happiness. This is the real, hidden beauty of your body: it is your greatest teacher and guide to a successful and fulfilling life.

The best way to answer the question *what is energy?* is, therefore, to first reveal the way—or all the different ways—it feels as it communicates information to you. Sometimes this can be the energy of inner happiness communicating the message, "Everything is okay, you're on the right track." Or it could be the energy of discomfort communicating the message, "You need to sort something out before being able to continue on the right track." Whatever you feel in your body has a message for you. Once you have experienced all the ways energy can feel, the ways you experience it, then you will know what it is. And when you know it, you can then begin to read it, to interpret it. It's like learning a new language, only this language is that of your body.

## My First Experience of Subtle Energy

My first direct experience of subtle energy occurred in November 2002, in Chiang Mai, Northern Thailand, when I received a Thai massage treatment from Chaiyuth Priyasith, regarded by many as one of the greatest living masters of Thai massage. Chaiyuth was a deeply spiritual man and a devout Buddhist. He loved the Lord Buddha and offered daily prayers and thanks to him, as well as to his beloved Shivago Komarpaj, the accredited founding figure of Thai medicine, and to Kruba Srivichai, a highly revered monk of Chiang Mai. Chaiyuth was also deeply involved in local shamanism and regularly attended ritual spirit dances during which ancestral spirits would be conjured and made manifest in particular dancers through channeling and possession. This was the magic of Thai massage in Chiang Mai—it was a combination of body work, Buddhist spirituality, and shamanic energy.

At the time, Chaiyuth's reputation as a healer and somewhat of a magician in Thai massage was the stuff of legend. A massage from him lasted anywhere between three and seven hours, and it was said he was able to regrow dead internal organs or revitalize a person's entire energy system in a single treatment. For these reasons, the prospect of receiving a treatment from this great master was very exciting to me, and I eagerly anticipated my afternoon appointment.

It was a warm, sunny day, and Chaiyuth was in full flow. As usual, he worked with his eyes closed, seemingly in a trance. Around thirty minutes into the massage, I began to feel cold—not cold from the outside, but rather cold from the inside. I began to shake and shiver. I developed goosebumps and my hair stood on end. I thought it very odd to be feeling so cold when it was sunny and 86 degrees on the veranda of his house where the massage took place. I began to lose control of my breathing and soon became very uncomfortable. This was not what I was expecting! By the end of the treatment I was soaking wet, cold, and exhausted. I also felt like I weighed about 250 pounds. It took me fifteen minutes to get up off the floor. I said nothing. I couldn't—I didn't have the energy to speak. So I just left.

I stumbled back to the guesthouse where I was staying. The otherwise short journey took over an hour, as I had to sit down and gather myself after every twenty or so steps. I was completely disoriented. That was late on a Tuesday afternoon. I spent all day Wednesday and Thursday shaking and sweating, unable to eat anything. On Friday morning I finally threw up, after which everything magically settled and I felt normal again. I returned to Chaiyuth and asked him what had happened. In his usual cryptic and playful manner, he replied, "You closed, now you open." I knew straightaway he was referring to energy, but it was only later that I fully understood what had actually happened in the treatment, and how common a reaction like this can be in any process of healing or self-development, not only in Thai massage.

Chaiyuth had worked with me on a level much deeper than what happens during the average massage. He worked through my physical body into my energetic body and found in me an energy that was prevalent throughout much of my life: the energy of fear. The entire massage he gave me was nothing more than a movement and a flow of fear energy within my body. This was my first real experience of subtle-body energy. The fundamental thing I learned from this experience was that you first have to physically experience subtle energy before you can understand it and recognize it in yourself or in another person. What I experienced in this massage with Chaiyuth was the different ways in which the energy of fear can manifest as it is released from deep within the physical body. I learned what each manifestation feels like and, by extension, what signs to look for when the energy of fear releases into the body of someone else, whether a massage client or a student of yoga, meditation, or martial arts who is undertaking an intense practice.

Apart from generating the feeling of fear itself, the energy of fear also has a number of other metaphysical characteristics, including internal coldness, shivering, heaviness, sudden tiredness, sleepiness, irregular breathing, cold sweating, anxiety, loss of skin color, loss of energy, loss of appetite, inability to speak, inability to look another in the eye, dehydration, and nausea. It is also interesting to see how the triggering or activating of a particular energy can continue long after the trigger event itself has ended. This is why someone can feel unsettled for a few days after a particularly strong experience, such as following an intense yoga, massage, or meditation retreat.

Prior to my massage with Chaiyuth, I had heard of fear. I knew what it was and what it could do to you, but I had never felt its true physical essence, not until that day. Now that I had felt it and experienced it, I was able to understand it, describe it, and use this knowledge in my massage practice and in my own personal self-development. This is how it works with energy. You first have to touch it and experience it. Then you absorb the experience and learn all about it, and only then can you integrate that knowledge into your life.

It is not necessary to travel all the way to Thailand and receive a massage from a master in order to experience the energy of your body; you can do it wherever you are and at any time that is convenient for you. Some readers may have already experienced the physiological effects of subtle-body energy, whether through yoga, massage, meditation, tai chi, or any other practice that involves the movement of subtle energy. If you have not, don't worry. It's easy to do. The best way to start is to find a partner with whom you can spend some time and with whom you can do some simple hands-on and hands-off energy exercises.

### Your Natural Sensitivity to Energy

Some people naturally have a greater sensitivity to energy. They see colors, they can read auras, they receive intuitive messages, etc. When they touch you, they can somehow easily read you and can be intuitively drawn to the parts of your body that need healing or treatment. You could say they are naturally gifted healers. I'm not one of these people.

When I first learned Thai massage in London with my teachers

Amy Ku Redler and Andrea Baglioni, I had all the sensitivity of a concrete brick. Things are different now. I developed my sensitivity to energy through years of massage practice, but initially through the work I did with my energy teacher in Chiang Mai, Jasmine Vishnu. Working with Jasmine, I found that by developing sensitivity to my own energy I somehow became equally sensitive to the energy of my clients. For instance, as I explored, or processed, the energies held in my low back, pelvic girdle, and upper thighs, a body area roughly corresponding to the area of the root chakra, I became more sensitive to and understanding of the same energies clients held in their root chakra. Over the years I explored energies held in many parts of my body, and as I did so I became more sensitive to and understanding of the energies held in the same body parts of my clients. This meant I was better able to understand the nature of the energy or energy blockage in my clients and so was better able to help people process, understand, and release that energy.

If you are interested in energy work in massage, don't worry if you don't have any sensitivity to energy. You can develop sensitivity to energy through the examination of your own energy system using the services of an energy teacher or spiritual teacher or through the naturally developing sensitivity to energy that comes from regular massage practice. It's the way most of us do it.

## Exploring Subtle Energy with a Partner

One of the best ways to begin tuning in to the subtle energy of the body is to partner up with someone you know, perhaps a fellow massage or yoga practitioner, and give him or her a little foot massage. It's best to do this on the floor. Ask your partner to lie down on a massage or yoga mat while you kneel down between the person's feet. Your partner can remain fully clothed for this exercise (but should remove socks). Don't worry if you have never massaged anyone before. This exercise is easy. Start out by resting your hands on your partner's feet, with your thumbs on the soles of the feet and your fingers on the dorsa. Just touch and hold the feet for a while, then squeeze them gently. Rub and massage them if you wish. What do you feel? You can do both feet at the same time or one at a time, it doesn't matter.

The first thing you will probably notice about the person's feet is whether they feel warm or cold. They may also feel hard or soft. What about the skin? It might feel a bit wet, or spongy, or even sticky. Alternatively it may feel dry. When you squeeze a foot, is the area you squeeze yielding to your touch? Is the foot soft, like butter, or harder, like a piece of wood wrapped in soft leather? Maybe the sole of the foot is soft, but the dorsum is hard, or vice versa. If you massage both feet at the same time, you may find one feels different than the other—this is not uncommon. Although you may not yet realize it, when you tune in to the qualities of your partner's feet, you are actually connecting with and reading the subtle energy in the body of the person. What you notice are subtle indications as to the overall health of the person:

### Healthy Feet, Healthy Energy

Feet that feel dry, soft, and yielding to the touch are a sign of healthy feet. Indeed, any body area that is normally warm and normally dry to the touch and is soft and yielding is a sign of good health in that particular part of the body. On the other hand, feet that are hard, spongy, wet, or sticky reveal an imbalance in subtle-body energy. A body area that feels spongy to the touch indicates a strong presence of water energy, also known as yin, female, or second-chakra energy. An example can be seen in women who present with spongy ankles, feet, or hands during menstruation; the spongy or slightly swollen feeling indicates a strong release of water energy into the system, which in the case of a menstruating woman will pass after a few days.

### Wet Feet, Wet Energy

Feet that are wet indicate a strong presence of yin, water, or second-chakra energy; wet, normal temperature, and soft feet indicate the presence of strong, positive yin, female energy. Wet, hot, and soft feet indicate the presence of very strong, positive yin, female energy. They may also indicate an ongoing process of detoxification, as often follows a visit to a Native American sweatlodge. Wet, cold, and soft feet indicate the presence of a cold energy, such as loneliness or fear. Wet, cold, and hard feet indicate the strong presence of cold energy, the hardness indicating the person's inability to let go of the cold energy causing the blockage.

### Sticky Feet, Sticky Energy

Feet that are sticky indicate the presence of a correspondingly sticky energy such as fear or insecurity. Sticky, normal temperature, and soft feet indicate a low-level presence of insecurity or fear. Sticky, cold, hard feet indicate a strong presence of insecurity or fear. It should be noted that the insecurity, which is a very sticky energy, may not be the insecurity of the person whose feet you are touching, but alternatively the insecurity of another person sticking to the person. If, for example, your mother is feeling insecure and takes shelter from her feelings by spending time with you, she will pass on the energy of her insecurity to you. It can be quite hard to release this kind of energy, because, as in real life, when an insecure person finds a place where they feel safe and secure, it can be difficult to extract that person from that place. Be aware that when you encounter the energy of insecurity in the body of a person, that energy will tend to stick to your own hands. Fear is another kind of sticky energy, and as a sticky energy it attracts other energies to itself. This is the root of the often-asked question, "Why do I always attract the very things I am afraid of?" This is because the energy of fear attracts in kind when projected. If you are a massage therapist, it can be useful to have a saucer in your massage room with a few lit tea lights on it, so that if you ever feel your hands becoming sticky during a massage, you can hold them over the candle flames until you feel the stickiness burn off and your hands becoming dry.

### Cool to Cold Energy

There is an important difference between cool and cold energy when it comes to forming a diagnosis of the energetic condition of a person. Cool energy is normal and healthy, whereas cold represents a blockage. One of the best ways to tell the difference between cool and cold is that an area of body tissue containing cool energy will be soft and yielding to the touch, whereas a body area containing cold energy will feel dense, heavy, hard, and unyielding. A great part of the body on which to test this is the calf muscle. When you squeeze a calf muscle containing cool energy, you will be able to squeeze all the way through the soft muscle tissue. You should also be able to form an *O* with your grip, with your thumb and fingers meeting in the space between muscle and bone. You should also be able to lift the calf muscle away from the bone. When you squeeze a calf muscle containing cold energy, you will only be able to generate medium pressure with your hand before finding muscular resistance or density. You will not be able to feel the softness of the muscle tissue. In severe cases, the calf muscle will feel as hard as wood, or when you squeeze it gently it will feel as if there is a piece of semisolid ice under the skin's surface.

Cool energy is yin, water, female energy. It can also be the energy used in sexual healing. It is soft black in color and represents energy in a natural, neutral, healthy state. Cold energy, on the other hand, is generally related to some form of life hurt and is the opposite of the warmth and openness of the heart. Some of the most commonly found cold energies include loneliness, lovelessness (if you were conceived in lovelessness, there will be ice-cold energy in your navel), grief, sadness, despair, fear, self-doubt, and lack of self-love. The deeper the condition, the more icy the temperature of the energy and the more dense, heavy, or contracted the body tissue in the area close to where the cold energy is stored, for example, at the top of the hamstrings where the experience of childhood loneliness is stored in the body.

Anesthesia used during a dental or surgical procedure releases enormous coldness into the body as its effectiveness fades. The release of physical pain from an area of hurt in the body also releases coldness into the body.

### Dry Skin, Dry Energy
An area of the body where the skin is very dry and feels flaky, cracked, crusty, or is broken and weeping also indicates an excessive buildup of

subtle-body energy leading to a blockage in the flow of a particular energy, in this example, fire energy. The skin often appears pinkish red in color and can be very sensitive to any kind of contact. Even touching the area with your hand can cause irritation. Fire describes the energy belonging to the heart area of the body, an area also referred to as the heart chakra, or fourth chakra.

### Feeling the Energy of a Chakra

Now that you have your partner feeling all relaxed after your wonderful foot massage, you can do a second exercise.

Ask your partner to remain where she is. Kneel down alongside her torso with your pelvis roughly in line with her pelvis. Face toward her head. Make sure the air around her body is still. Using one hand, held an inch or two over your partner's body, scan her body to see if you can sense areas that feel hot or areas that feel cold. If you find you're not picking up on anything, use your other hand, as you may find that one of your hands is better at sensing energy than the other. After a while, you may begin to discern three things: the areas of your partner's body that feel normal in temperature, the areas that feel colder than normal, and the areas that feel hotter than normal. You can also use visual aids to help you with your diagnosis. The skin color of body areas that feel hotter than normal tend to appear reddish. Those areas that are cold tend to look pale, gray, or white.

What is interesting to note is that although you may feel that certain areas of your partner's body are hotter or colder than normal, the person's actual body temperature does not vary. This may seem like a contradiction but it is not. There are two things a thermometer does not measure when measuring body temperature: the flow of energy running through the area of the body where the thermometer is placed, and the degree of emotional energy in the body area where the thermometer is placed. An area of the body through which there is a high degree of energy moving will feel hotter to your hand than normal, whereas a body area through which there is a very low degree of energy running will feel cooler. In both cases a thermometer reading will show no variation in body temperature.

You may additionally experience a slight buzzing on your hand, a tickling, a tingling feeling, or what some people refer to as "a feeling of ants on my skin." Alternatively, you may feel something like needles or pulsing in your hand. These are all signs that your hand is tuning in to and sensing the subtle energy in the body of your practice partner.

You may also feel a very slight pressure under your hand when held over certain areas of your partner's body, like a magnetic field. It may feel like an invisible soft, spongy ball. You may feel that the pressure causes your hand to be pushed away from your partner's body, or alternatively, you may feel your hand being pulled in toward the person's body. Both these sensations relate to areas in the body where energy is either expanding or contracting. You may even feel that your hand is being pulled or pushed to the left or right or in a slightly circular movement, either clockwise or counterclockwise. This indicates you are discovering the strong energy centers known as *chakras* (discussed in greater detail in chapter 2). Finally, you may feel something like an invisible tube, or a funnel, a vortex, or a cone under your hand. All these sensations, from a tingling on the palm of your hand to your hand being turned in a circular direction, are indications that you are tuning in to the subtle energy in your partner's body—the same energy you have in your own body, energy that you are, for the most part, normally unaware of or cannot feel, yet energy that has a significant impact on the physical condition of the body.

Emotional energy, which we will explore in greater detail in chapter 3, plays a significant role in how hot or cold certain areas of the body feel. Emotions, or emotional energy, have variations in temperature. Some emotions feel cold, like fear, while others feel hot, like love. If you hold your hand over a part of your partner's body where she is holding the energy of fear, you will feel a small area of cold in the center of the palm of your hand, whereas the energy of love will feel hot on your hand. Similarly if you suddenly feel cold during a massage or yoga practice, it may reveal that a cold emotional energy, such as grief or fear, is being released into your body. Fear, which is a water energy, not only causes you to feel cold when released but, because water is heavy, can also leave you feeling heavy. You may not experience fear directly because the energy release is too small to give rise to the actual emotion, but the release is big enough for you to notice the effect it is having in your body.

Feelings of buzzing on your hand, coldness, hardness of the person's feet, or wetness on the person's skin are all experiences of subtle energy. For many, these are the first experiences of subtle-body energy and can be easily found when doing the two simple exercises described above. Some people, however, have different experiences when doing these exercises. They may see colors or images in their mind; others may experience empathetic feelings in their own body, like agitation, a headache, or a tightness in the abdomen. These are all legitimate experiences of subtle energy and show us that some people have different ways of experiencing and interpreting this energy. This is the main reason why I cannot tell my students precisely what they will experience when they look for subtle energy. Yes, it may be so for some people, but for others it may be something completely different. We are all of us unique in the ways we connect to and communicate with everything around us, including the energy of our body and the energy of a partner's body. This is why anyone interested in energy has to experience it for themselves, by themselves, in order to discover their own unique way of reading energy and their own personal vocabulary of terms of how to describe their findings.

Don't be concerned if at first you don't see colors in your mind's eye when you do these exercises; if you keep practicing you soon will. Similarly, don't be concerned if you feel nothing at all when you first attempt these exercises. There are lots of reasons for this happening. Maybe your partner is too relaxed, and you are not relaxed enough. Give it a couple of goes, and all will be revealed. I have never encountered anyone who is genuinely interested in exploring subtle energy who did not eventually discover how to see it.

## Other Ways of Detecting Subtle Energy

### Pain

Pain is a common manifestation of subtle energy, or, to be more precise, a manifestation of a blockage in subtle energy, although not all forms of pain indicate an energy blockage. There is a simple way to tell the difference between regular pain and pain that is caused by a blockage in the body's subtle energy. If you find you have a pain in a particular part of your body, see if you can pinpoint the pain by touching it with your index finger. If the pain is ordinary pain, as soon as you touch the spot you will let out an "Ow!" This is pain of specific physiological origin, for example, a cut or a bruise to the skin, a torn or ruptured muscle or ligament, an inflammation or swelling caused by an infection. It's something that hurts the moment you touch it.

Pain caused by an energy blockage is harder to pinpoint; it is something beyond touch. When you try to pinpoint it, you may find it difficult to do so. You may feel that the pain is deeper inside, beyond your touch. You may even feel that you have a physical pain in a part of your body, such as your lower back, yet when you touch the area your touch does not cause any pain. It is almost as if when you touch the pain, the pain vanishes. This is not a trick on the part of your body; rather, this reveals an area of your body that is reacting to a blockage in subtle energy that lies just off the surface of your skin. It is the same as holding your hand over a naked flame; you feel the pain on the skin of your hand, but the source of the pain lies away from the surface of your skin.

Pain caused by a blockage in your subtle energy is the kind of pain that doesn't show up in X-rays or in ultrasound tests or scans. It is a pain your general practitioner cannot diagnose, yet to you it is legitimate and real. It is a pain that can last days, weeks, months, or even years, and then mysteriously vanish, leaving no physical damage. Sometimes it is sudden and sharp, sometimes dull and long-lasting. It is pain without rules. If you have this type of pain, you are dealing with a blockage in your subtle energy.

### Tension

Tension is another manifestation of subtle energy that can be easily felt in the body. Tension, although it tends to have a negative connotation, is not always a bad thing. The release of energy through the muscles, internal organs, or connective tissue naturally creates a temporary flux or tension, creating resistance, but not tightness or hardness. This is why a person can sometimes feel a stiffness or resistance to movement the morning after a massage. This kind of stiffness indicates an ongoing release of blocked energy. When the release subsides, so does the feeling of stiffness. It's a natural process.

Tension can also indicate the presence of an acute or chronic blockage in subtle energy. In massage, you may encounter a person who comes to you after having had a bad week at work and is seething with frustration over something. You can feel the buzz or vibration of this energy as soon as you touch the person. You may also have a client who is carrying a long-term chronic medical condition, or who has been on a long-term regime of heavy medication. Both situations can create tension that you can feel in yourself or in the body of the person as a tension that is held deeper in the body. This kind of tension is a little finer and less aggressive than the "seething with rage" type of tension.

In massage, there is no single approach to treating tension. You may have two seething-with-rage clients in one day who require very different styles of treatment, one vigorous, one gentle. Tension needs to be dealt with on a case-by-case basis, and appropriate treatment is something you learn only through personal experience and practice. That's the way it is. Some people respond better to gentle touch, while others respond better to a more vigorous touch. The only way to find out is to play around with it. If you have a client with tight muscles in the lower back, for instance, see if the muscles respond better to a slow, gentle, warming touch, or to a more pointed, vigorous touch. Be guided by what you feel. Don't be concerned if you end up using gentle touch and the person says he feels nothing. There are times in massage when what the person feels you are doing is very different from what you know you are doing. If you feel the muscles relax with gentle touch, then you are doing the right thing.

### *Abstract Manifestations of Subtle Energy*

Here are some deeper, more subtle expressions of subtle-body energy that are not as easily noticed as pain or tension.

## Spasms, Involuntary Jerking, Cramping (Feet or Hands), Catatonia
These are examples of an acute movement or release of energy held in a chakra, meridian, internal organ, muscle, or nerve.

## Lumps or Clots
These are small, semisoft lumps of coagulated energy just under the skin surface. They feel like blood clots but are not and dissolve after light massaging. They tend to be in area of the abdomen and calf muscles.

## An Inability to Look Someone Directly in the Eye
This reveals the strong presence of a second-chakra emotional energy, fear, in the body of the person unable to make eye contact.

## An Inability to Maintain Eye Contact
This reveals a strong release of third-chakra energy into the body, causing heightened agitation and the inability to remain still enough to maintain eye contact.

## Intense Eye Contact
This indicates a person who is unable to ground their energy through their own body due to a blockage in the first chakra and so needs to ground their energy through you.

## Restlessness
This indicates a strong release of second- or third-chakra energy into the body, causing unease or agitation.

## Heaviness
Sometimes in massage when you lift a person's leg it feels heavier or lighter than expected—an indication of a blockage in energy. If it feels heavier than expected, this is a manifestation of an excess of heavy first- and second-chakra energies that the person has been unable to ground or let go of through their lower legs and feet. If lighter than expected, this reveals a blockage in the area of the anterior inferior iliac spine (or AIIS, the bony eminence on the anterior border of the hip bone, or,

more precisely, the wing of the ilium), stopping energy flowing downward into the legs. The leg is empty of energy and therefore feels light.

Note that the same heaviness effect can be observed when you give someone a massage that focuses mostly on the legs and lower torso. The client can feel heavy following such a treatment. Conversely, when you give a massage to someone in which the focus of the session is on the upper half of the torso, the client can leave feeling light, or lightheaded. This is because the energy housed in the two lowest energy centers of the body, the first and second chakras, is said to be heavier than the energies housed in the higher chakras. There is no scientific proof of this phenomenon, but just ask anyone how they feel after a strong leg massage and they will most likely say "heavy."

Also note that sometimes a client's leg can feel light when you lift it because the person is lifting the leg for you, which can happen when the person is stressed and unable to relax. As the energy of stress is housed in the third chakra, the person who unconsciously lifts her leg for you in a massage is revealing an imbalance, or excess, of third-chakra energy.

Meditation, by the way, provides us with another opportunity for noting the difference between heavy and light energy. Dynamic forms of meditation, such as OSHO Dynamic Meditation, that include lots of movement, dancing, or stamping on the floor are necessary to vitalize the heavier energies of the first two chakras, including kundalini energy, which is housed at the base of the second chakra. On the other hand, in a sitting meditation practice like Vipassana, no movement is required to vitalize the higher, spiritual energies of the fifth and sixth chakras, where less physical work is needed to move these lighter forms of energy.

## Tiredness

Feeling continuously tired when you have no reason to be, when you are otherwise eating well, sleeping well, and work is going well, can be indicative of an imbalance in an aspect of your current lifestyle. This could relate to the fact that a) you are in the wrong place; b) you are doing the wrong thing; or c) you are with the wrong person or people. "Wrong" in this case means that where you are, who you are with, or what you are doing is not serving your best or highest purpose. It is time to move on. Your spirit is bored, hence the fatigue.

## Sudden Tiredness When You Have No Reason to Be, Most Notably at Night

This can indicate the presence of a high-vibration energy, or spirit, wishing to enter your energy field. As a massage therapist, yoga teacher or practitioner, energy worker, or channeler, you may also find that working with higher-vibration energies makes you tired.

## Sudden Localized Physical Weakness

Unexpected or inexplicable sudden physical weakness in joints or muscles, most typically in ankles, knees, lower back (between L5 and S1), upper arms, wrists, or elbows, can be indicative of energy blockages that will be discussed in detail when we explore thirty of the most common energetic ailments in chapter 8.

## Sudden Sensitivity to Certain Foods, such as Dairy, Fried Foods, or Alcohol

In many instances, sensitivity to certain food types, or the inability to digest certain food types, reflects disharmony in the energies of the stomach and the spleen. The food itself is not causing the person to feel sick but is an indicator of an already present underlying energy imbalance or disharmony, which is causing internal unease. This can happen, for example, when someone or some situation in your life is having too strong an effect on you. If you find yourself in a situation that is overbearing, or "hard to stomach," such as a domestic situation (in relation to a parent, sibling, child, spouse), a situation with a current or past partner, or a social situation (employer, colleague, friend, schoolmate), your body's energy system will reduce the amount of energy you take in from that situation or person in order to protect you from the energy of the person or situation. The limitation your body puts on the range of energy you ingest and digest from that situation is then reflected in the limitation it puts on the range of energy you are normally able to ingest and digest from another important energy source: food.

The energy you use for self-protection originates in the spleen. One of the normal functions of the spleen is to provide heating energy for the stomach to help it digest food effectively. But if some of that energy is diverted for the purpose of self-protection, than less energy is diverted to the stomach, making the stomach less able to properly digest. Sometimes the cure for food sensitivity is not to control or limit your diet but to investigate your environment and see if there is anything that is having an overbearing effect on you. This may be a person who has been in your life for a long time, for example, a parent or spouse. However, as it is in life, it is easier to blame food for this type of discomfort than it is to look closely at your life and the people in it.

## Energy Blockages

An energy blockage is an accumulation of subtle-body energy from current or former sources that has become stored in a particular part of the body. It's a bit like the accumulation and storage of fat in the body; whereas fat is a solidified form of nutritional energy, an energy blockage is the metaphysical solidification in the body of negative experiences of the eight types of subtle energy, as shown in the following examples.

**Emotional Energy,** such as grief, fear, anger, jealousy

**Mental Energy,** such as the unwillingness let go, the need to dominate people, or the refusal to forgive someone who has hurt you

**Sexual Energy,** such as the use of sex to fill a void or forced or coerced sex

**Karmic Energy,** such as the energy of your own past lives that comes back to you in your current life

**Spiritual Energy,** such as a distorted sense of truth or lack of access to higher intellect and consciousness

**Environmental Energy,** such as stress at work or home

**Interpersonal Energy,** such as your partner, colleague, or teacher taking his or her anger out on you

**Ancestral Energy,** such as unreleased negative experiences in your parents' lives, which are passed on to you at the time of your conception; ancestral energy can also include generations further back, such as grandparents or great-grandparents, who pass along energy patterns to succeeding generations

An energy blockage can result from an traumatic event, such as the shock at being robbed or mugged; or it can be the result of a long-term chronic situation, such as living in an environment where you are constantly afraid of a spouse or a parent.

Under normal circumstances, the body is able to process and let go of a certain amount of harmful subtle energy, just as it is able to ingest, digest, and evacuate a certain amount of harmful nutritional energy such as junk food. But if we ingest too much harmful food—for example, greasy chips or fast food—the body eventually becomes unable to digest and evacuate all of the unhealthy grease and toxic ingredients properly, so the remainder of it gets sent to a part of the body for storage. While the body stores unprocessed food as fat, it stores unprocessed subtle energy as an energy blockage.

Say you work in a frustrating business environment. Under normal, day-to-day circumstances your body is able to process and release low levels of frustration energy. Sometimes if the level of frustration at work rises, you may find a need to do some form of physical activity, like going to the gym or running, to help the body burn off and get rid of this energy. From time to time, however, you might have a really bad day at the office, during which you get so frustrated that your body is simply unable to process and release all of the negative energy. On such occasions, the excess energy of frustration that your body is unable to process gets pushed down and stored in some part of your body. Now imagine you have been working in a constantly frustrating work environment for the last ten years. Add up the effects of all those bad days when you were unable to process and get rid of your frustration, and you will begin to see how an energy blockage can develop. It might not have felt like much to you ten years ago, but all this frustration has been slowly, subtly building up inside you until you now find yourself in a semipermanent state of poor sleep, low-level agitation, quick temperedness, shoulder and chest tightness, breathing irregularities, sensitivity to certain food types, and an inability to find peace of mind. These conditions are all characterstic of an energy blockage.

In most instances energy blockages in the body go largely unnoticed; however, some energy blockages become large enough to take on physiological characteristics. Some of the more common symptoms of energy blockage in the body include sticky skin, a feeling of cold in the abdomen, tightening muscles, nonspecific body pain, excessive tiredness, inflammation in the neck, headache, and sensitivity to certain foods.

### Mental Energy

Of all the different classifications of subtle energy, mental energy is the most difficult to describe fully, as its scope is so wide. Mental energy is the energy that gives rise to all aspects of idea, thought, belief, judgment, decision-making, planning, will, execution, and resolution. It also governs learning, memory and recollection, evolved patterns of personal and social behavior, all the emotions that feed into anger, and, of course, all aspects of mental illness and imbalance.

Much of this book details different types of subtle energy, such as the different emotions or the different types of sexual energy. But as this is practically impossible to do for mental activity, discussion of mental energy is mostly limited to its physical and metaphysical effects on the body. This is detailed in chapter 2 in the discussion of the third chakra, the center of mental energy in the body. Additional references to third-chakra energy, and therefore by extension mental energy, are to be found throughout the book.

## Energy Blocks

An energy block occurs when what starts as an energy blockage is further compounded by a conscious decision to take no action to address the blockage.

Not forgiving your parents for giving you a tough start in life creates an energy block. It takes a lot of mental energy to continually not forgive someone over a period of years. This causes a huge buildup of mental energy in the body, creating tension and hardness in certain parts of the body as well as causing great hurt to another part of the body, the heart, the nature of which is to forgive and let go. Knowing that your unwillingness to forgive and let go is causing you pain in certain parts of your body—for instance your arms, chest, heart, or other organs—and then making the conscious decision to do nothing about it puts a block on the energy blockage ever being released.

To summarize, energy blockages originate from any one of eight types of subtle energy: emotional, mental, sexual, spiritual, environmental, interpersonal, ancestral, and karmic. In general all emotional, mental, and ancestral energies originate in the first, second, and third chakras. Later in this book we'll consider what each of these eight types of energies feels like in the body and, by extension, what a corresponding blockage in that particular energy feels like. Although the presence of any kind of energy blockage or block can have an adverse effect on the physical condition of the body, the good news is that nothing is irrevocable; blockages, and even long-held blocks, for that matter, can be undone and released from the body, oftentimes through a form of therapy or recovery that includes some form of free-form physical movement that addresses the energy of the body. A mixture of yoga, walking in nature, free-form dancing, and meditation makes for a good combination.

# 2

# Energy Balancing in
# the Chakras and Meridians

A chakra is an opening or wormhole* in the body that draws in energy from the environment and distributes it, via energy channels, or in traditional Chinese medicine (TCM) the energy meridians, throughout the physical body. Chakras and their energies are invisible to ordinary eyes, but some people who are sensitive to energy or who have been trained to have extended sight, such as clairvoyants or energy workers, can see them as areas or streams of colored light.

The energies drawn in by the chakras feed our emotional, mental, and spiritual needs during certain stages of development in life. In the stage of infancy, for example, a newborn needs the energies of welcome, reward, and parental love in order to develop feelings of self-identity, self-worth, and trust. These energies enter the body of the infant through the root chakra. More about these kinds of developmental needs as they relate to the different chakras later in this chapter . . .

If all our needs relating to a certain developmental stage in life are

---

*A highly stylized interpretation of a chakra can be seen during the opening credits of the *Star Trek: Deep Space Nine* TV show (available on YouTube), in which a normally invisible wormhole opens out in a circular movement to allow traffic—i.e., energy—to pass through in both directions.

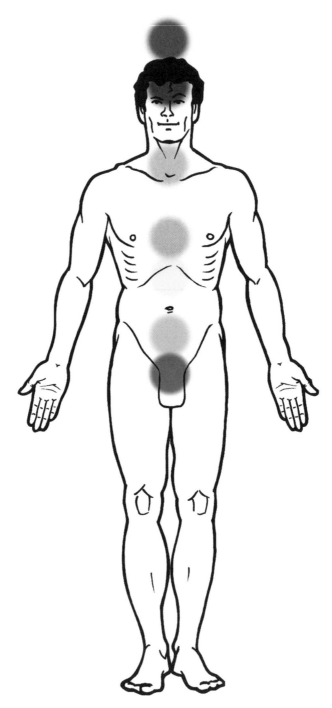

*Fig. 2.1. The chakras*

met, the energy housed in the chakra relating to that stage of development is said to be balanced. If not, then it is said that there is an unfulfilled energetic need in the chakra. A chakra with an unfulfilled energetic need will continue to draw energy to itself well beyond its related life-developmental stage in an attempt to make itself fulfilled. For example, an adult who does not remember his unfulfilled needs during infancy, which are mirrored in the energetic condition of his first chakra, will subconsciously try to draw energy from his environment in an attempt to fulfill the energetic void in this chakra. This might include the energy of pleasure (a second-chakra energy), the energy of emotional love (a fourth-chakra energy), the energy of security that comes from the accumulation of wealth (a third-chakra energy), or the energy of spiritual love (a sixth-chakra energy). Some massage therapists or yoga teachers, for example, subconsciously try to replace their unfulfilled energetic need for parental love during infancy with the energy of love that comes from massage clients or yoga students. For some adults, the subconscious need to fulfill a forgotten, unmet childhood need can be the root of addiction; for others, it can drive them to great achievements.

Although environmental energies such as love, support, and reward are different from the energies the body receives from food, water, air, or sunshine, which relate directly to the physiological development of the body, the quality of environmental energy that forms the energy in the chakras nevertheless has an impact on one's physiological development and the condition of the body. For instance, an infant born into a cold and unloving environment will protect herself from this cold and unloving energy. She does this by drawing into herself and contracting or closing her body against the coldness around her. This action of protection is mirrored in the condition of certain parts of her physical body, which also become contracted and turned away as she develops, such as contracted or tight muscles in the lower back, pelvis, and hamstrings. Even the pelvis itself can become turned away or tilted on its axis. These physical conditions, which reflect unfulfilled energetic needs in the first and second chakras, are often carried into adulthood, although their origins are long forgotten. The proper course of action for opening and releasing such bodily conditions involves addressing the underlying energetic needs of the first and second chakras and fulfilling those needs. Attempting to open or release tight, contracted, or twisted muscles without reference to their energetic origins in the person's early environment may bring about only a partial release. Repeated attempts to release tight or contracted muscles without such reference could even lead to additional physical problems.

That environmental energies can bring about an adverse effect on the physical body is not only a factor of earliest childhood experiences; this kind of influence can come into play later in adulthood. For example, as adults, we tend to close ourselves off to the threatening emotional or mental energies of a stressful work environment. This action of self-protection is mirrored in a tightening in certain areas of the body, especially in the shoulders, neck, midback, and digestive system. The energies in a stressful work environment enter the body through the third chakra, located in the solar plexus, and are distributed throughout the body along the meridians associated with the third chakra: the liver, gallbladder, stomach, and spleen meridians. This is why the physiological effects of stress on the body can be so pervasive.

## Anatomy of a Chakra

Although there are numerous chakras in the subtle body according to ancient yogic and tantric texts, there are seven major chakras considered to be the most important ones. Each is related to a specific stage of development in life:

**First chakra:** Environmental needs around the time of our birth and earliest childhood

**Second chakra:** Environmental needs when we start to build a sense-based understanding of our world

**Third chakra:** Environmental needs when we start to build a rational, intellectual-based understanding of our world

**Fourth chakra:** Our understanding of love and how we give and receive love in adulthood

**Fifth chakra:** Our need for a more truthful understanding of our world

**Sixth chakra:** Our need for a spiritual understanding of our world

**Seventh chakra:** The attainment of a full understanding about our world, or enlightenment

Within each stage of development we need a range of different energies from our environment to fulfill the developmental needs at that particular stage of life. Different types of environmental energy have different levels of vibration, or frequency, and by extension give off different resonances in the form of different colors (color being a form of energy). In the earliest stage of life, for instance, we need a wide range of environmental energies, including maternal love, paternal love, a pleasant environment to live in, and a cuddly toy to squeeze or make us laugh. These different things in our environment feed us with different types of energy. Maternal love is a red energy, paternal love green, a cuddly toy orange, and a nice room to sleep in a yellow energy. These energies of different colors, or vibratory frequencies, enter our energy system through the energy center located in the root of the body, at the perineum.

In a similar way, each of the chakras houses different types of environmental energy, and these different types of energy have different colors, as seen in figure 2.1 on page 24. Accordingly, each chakra has a red layer, an orange layer, a yellow layer, a green layer, a sky blue layer, an indigo layer, and a purple layer. At the center of each chakra is a core of white light, which runs through our body and is the beam or ray of light that represents our spiritual identity. Each layer of similar color within each chakra is interconnected. So the layer of red energy in the first chakra is connected to the layer of red energy in the second chakra, in the third chakra, in the fourth chakra, and so on. The layer of orange energy in the first chakra is connected to the layer of orange energy in the second chakra, in the third chakra, in the fourth chakra, and so on. This type of interconnection applies to all the different layers of color within all seven chakras.

At the most basic level, the seven layers of color in a chakra represent the following:

**Layer 1, red:** The energy flowing between you and your family

**Layer 2, orange:** The energy that results from creativity, fun, and play in your life

**Layer 3, yellow:** Academic and intellectual energy; the energy of money

**Layer 4, green:** The amount of love energy in your life

**Layer 5, sky blue:** The amount of truth you know behind all your life circumstances

**Layer 6, indigo:** The energy that comes from the realm outside our three-dimensional reality

**Layer 7, purple:** The bridge to the divine within

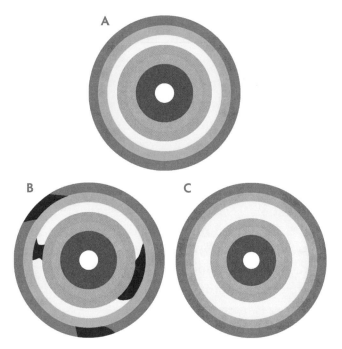

*Fig. 2.2. Representations of three chakra types (any of the seven individual chakras): (a) a balanced chakra; (b) a chakra with blockages in the red (familial) and yellow (intellectual) layers; (c) an imbalanced chakra with slight excess of yellow (intellectual) and slight lack of sky blue and indigo (metaphysical), revealing a person who has been brought up to respect science and academia and to place little importance on "unprovable" spiritual matters and intuition*

Although each chakra is comprised of seven layers of different-colored energy circling around a central core, each chakra has a governing color, as mentioned previously: red for the first chakra, orange for the second chakra, yellow for the third chakra, green for the fourth chakra, sky blue for the fifth chakra, indigo for the sixth chakra, and purple for the seventh chakra. The governing color of a chakra is determined by its basic function and needs. Let's go back to our example of the newborn, whose fundamental needs are to be welcomed into the world, to be given a sense of identity, and to be loved by its parents. These are red energies. The cuddly toy, an orange energy, and a nice room to sleep in, a yellow energy, are secondary and tertiary energies. Since the fundamental environmental needs of the first chakra are red energies, the governing color of the first chakra is red.

We'll return to this discussion of the colors and fundamental needs of each chakra later in this chapter.

Each chakra, when healthy and clear of all major blockages, is a source of vitality, energy, tingling, freedom, happiness, radiance, and love. Only when there is a blockage or some residual pain or something that needs to be addressed in a chakra are the natural feelings of energy and vitality missing or not flowing fully.

## The Pairings of the Chakras

Of the seven chakras, chakras one to six are twinned, or paired. These are our bodily chakras, the chakras that govern our life lessons on earth. They are the six that require balancing in order for the highest chakra to be opened. The seventh chakra, because it is not of the body nor of the earth needs no such balancing. Chakras one to three house our life experiences during the first twenty or so years of life. As those early experiences shape our later life experiences, their energies are twinned in the chakras that relate to our later life, chakras four to six. What we are taught about love in childhood becomes our understanding of love in adulthood. What we are taught about spiritual matters in childhood becomes how we interact with spirituality in adulthood. In this regard it can also be said that difficulties that arise in our later life are usually rooted in our early life. If we have a blockage in the fourth chakra, which houses our adult understanding of love, the root of that blockage is probably in the first chakra, where we were first introduced to love. If we have a blockage in the sixth chakra, which seeks the need of spiritual nourishment, the root of that blockage is probably in the third chakra, where we were first educated about spiritual matters.

- The first chakra is paired with the fourth chakra; red is paired with green.
- The second chakra is paired with the fifth chakra; orange is paired with sky blue.
- The third chakra is paired with the sixth chakra; yellow is paired with indigo.

The condition of the first chakra strongly influences the health of the fourth chakra. Everyone's first experience of love is the love they receive from their mother and from their father and from the atmosphere of love that exists between their mother and father in infancy. These experiences form the layers of red and green energy in the first chakra. As the first chakra is paired with the fourth chakra, the energies in the red and green layers of the first chakra are reproduced in the red and green layers of the fourth chakra. Although in infancy you do not understand what these types of love are, you grow accustomed to what they *feel* like and to what their energies feel like. So later in adulthood these early feelings of love form the basis of your understanding of what love is and what love should be. As a result, in adult relationships you subconsciously seek out the feelings of love that most closely match the feelings of love you first felt in infancy—they are, after all, your only understanding of what love is. For you, anything else simply isn't love. This is the classic example of the type of love energy in your first chakra determining the type of love energy your fourth chakra seeks from the outside world. This insight can be helpful if you are an adult experiencing a difference between the type of love relationship you would like to have and the type of adult love relationship you are subconsciously attracting.

The pairings of the chakras can be useful knowledge for massage therapists specializing in energy work and energy healing, as the healing of one chakra may involve the healing of its twinned chakra. Yoga teachers too may want to consider that if a student is having difficulty with a yoga posture relating to the fourth chakra, the root of the difficulty may lie in the first chakra. It may be useful, therefore, to pair yoga postures that focus on both chakras.

# The Seven Major Chakras

## *The First Chakra*

**Sanskrit name:** Muladhara
**Location:** Front, perineum; back, tailbone
**Color:** Red
**Element:** Stone
**Vital functions:** Connection to God; if this connection is unavailable, then connection to love, specifically, mother love; if unavailable, then connection to symbols of mother love, such as Mother Earth, nature, etc.; also represents connection to one's family and one's ancestors
**Symbols that appear in dreams and meditations:** Rock, stone, and concrete; things made of stone or concrete, such as a concrete house or a building carved out of stone; finding yourself sitting in the bottom of a pyramid or in the basement of a house; biblically, the rock on which the church is built
**Meridians:** Urinary bladder, conception vessel, governing vessel, sushumna (i.e., the nadi, or channel, that connects the root and crown chakras)
**Areas of the body:** Entire pelvic girdle, including all the sacral and L5 vertebrae; hips, legs, thighs, hamstrings, adductors, knees, ankles, and feet; bones

### Developmental Needs

These are best understood by looking at the things a human being needs from birth to about seven years of age.

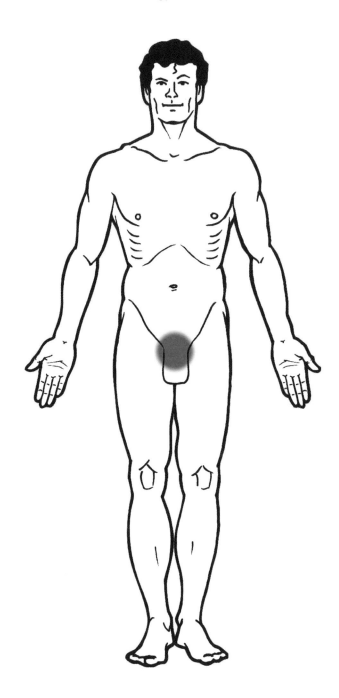

*Fig. 2.3. Location of the first chakra*

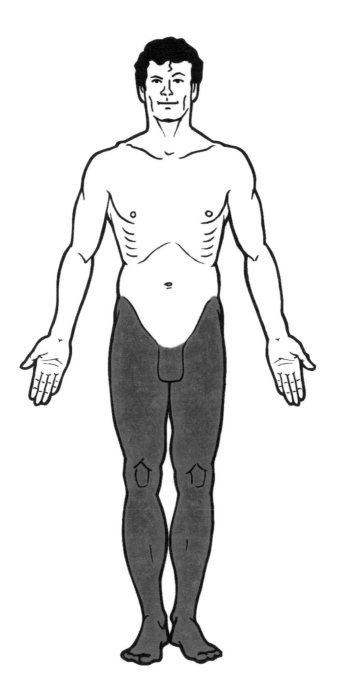

*Fig. 2.4. Area of the body governed by the first chakra (front)*

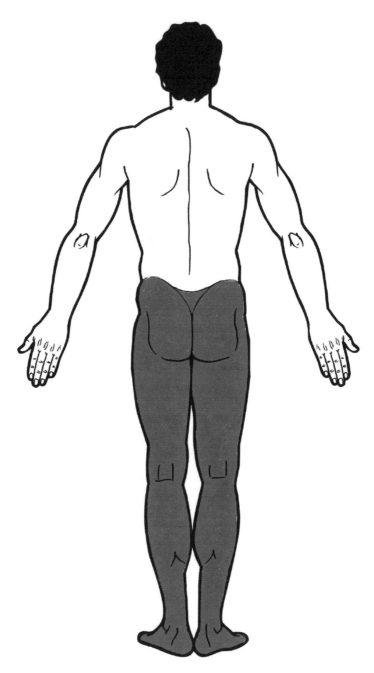

*Fig 2.5. Area of the body governed by the first chakra (back)*

Upon being born, the newborn needs to recognize where she is and that it is a happy and welcoming place. The quality of the energy of being welcomed into the world shapes the newborn's beliefs and, later in adulthood, the person's beliefs about the world as to whether it is overall a welcoming and happy place to be or a cold and hard place.

The infant needs to recover from birth and be *congratulated* for its efforts in being born. "Well done! Have a rest to recover. Here, lie on my belly, take as long as you need." This gives the fledgling person a sense of being understood. An infant not given sufficient time to rest and recover the energy lost from being born can experience heavy tiredness later as an adult.

The infant needs to be *rewarded* for its effort in being born. In the earliest stage of life, reward is best represented by food, and the best food you can give a child is milk from the breast. When you give a newborn the best possible reward, that child grows into adulthood knowing what is best for herself, having already experienced it. This will determine her ability to choose and decide what is best for her later in adult life, as she already has a deep understanding of what is best. Children not breast-fed tend to grow into adulthood having difficulty choosing what is best because they never learned what is best by getting the best. The other issue linked to not being breast-fed is unworthiness. Being given the bottle instead of the breast is, for the infant, to accept a substitution for what it really wants. This creates feelings of unworthiness that become the root of the feeling, later in adulthood, of not being worthy enough to ask for or get what you want—in other words, accepting second-best. People with unfulfilled childhood-reward needs will be driven to seek rewards throughout the rest of their adult lives, in other forms of energy such as the energy of pleasure. However, the sense of reward from the energy of pleasure cannot fill the void caused by unfulfilled reward energy at birth.

A newborn needs to be given *recognition* for who she is. Identifying expressions like "You're wonderful!" "You're our daughter (son)!" "You belong with us!" "You're a Henderson!" "You're Irish!" all carry a certain energetic quality, and this energy given to the child at birth determines the strength of the person's self-identity later in adulthood. This is the root of self-confidence.

A newborn needs to be *celebrated* for her efforts in being born. By doing this, the infant feels the energy of something being done for her or given to her, something celebratory, like a welcome-home party or a birthday party. This in turn forms the foundation of feelings of self-worth and support later in adulthood. A lack of this kind of celebration is the root of "I am worthless" or "I don't have the strength for this."

A newborn needs to be *heard*. When an infant cries, he is hungry and needs to be fed. The cry is the sound of the fledgling human being speaking his truth. If a person's needs are not heard when she speaks her truth from earliest life, the person grows into adulthood believing that no one listens to her. In such a case, she might try to find alternative ways of getting her "I need something" message across. The two most common alternative ways of saying "I need something" when you believe that no one listens to you when you speak your truth are lying and stealing. Conversely, being listened to is the root of trust in others and trust in life: "My needs will be met" and "The universe answers my needs."

A newborn needs to have his *wants* met. This is different from his needs. Whether it is extra food, rest, love, or reassurance, give a child what he wants. Newborns not given what they want grow up to be adults who do not know or are unable to get what they want in life. They can survive by fulfilling their basic needs but can never get what they want. It is as if there has never been room in their life for what they want.

The overall quality of *love* received in infancy determines the future adult's understanding of what love is and what their expectations of love are. The overall quality of love received in infancy refers to both the love between the child and the parents and the quality of love between the parents—the environmental energies that the child lives in and absorbs.

### What the Energy of the First Chakra Feels Like

As the energy of the first chakra is symbolized as stone, it is the heaviest of energies to move or to be moved, so there's a feeling of heaviness or weightiness associated with first-chakra energy. Feelings of shame, humiliation, repulsion, and disgust are all rooted in the first chakra. When you feel heavy or tired following a yoga practice or a massage, it can often be because you have been releasing and dealing with first-chakra energy. When vitalized and balanced, through yoga or massage, first-chakra energy gives rise to feelings of self-confidence, inner strength, power and purpose, trust and openness in life, and a sense of self-worth. Yoga postures associated with the first chakra include staff, bound angle, bridge, crab, half wind-relieving, full wind-relieving, locust, half warrior, and child's pose.

## Additional Functions

The first chakra also houses our karmic or past-life beliefs and experiences. These beliefs and experiences are subtle forms of energy that give shape to the circumstances in our earliest life and form the basis for the lessons we need to learn in this lifetime. Past lives are symbolic in form. Their stories offer deep insight into the roles of the conscious mind and the spiritual mind. What you see in your adult dreams of your past lives, such as you being a queen or a prisoner, are a symbolic retelling of a story from your current life. To dwell literally on a past life as an event that actually happened can lead to misunderstanding. You can end up believing in something that never happened, or doesn't exist.

The energy of the first chakra also has a smell, that of rotting flesh.

### Healing the First Chakra

It is possible in adulthood to undergo a healing of the first chakra's imbalances as a result of certain experiences missing from earliest childhood that are so necessary to the healthy development of this energy center. If your parents are still alive and if you still have a connection with them, working with your parents to help heal such hurts is the most effective form of first chakra healing. As this option, however, is not open to everyone, here are some additional ways to heal this chakra that do not require parental involvement:

**The Lady of the Lake** is a female persona who visits you in a dream or meditation and invites you to swim in a lake or pool she is protecting or guarding. The lake or pool is a symbol for the womb, and by entering it and swimming in it, you are offered the chance to be reborn. Its waters are either very dark or black. When you swim in this water, you experience the sheer bliss of rebirth, or being reborn the way you should have been born, filling you with everything you need for life. It is a healing of all the energies you swam in while in the womb of your mother. It reconnects you to the person you were born to be, the person you lost connection with due to the circumstances of the life you have lived so far. It is an incredibly beautiful experience. Upon emerging from the water the guardian figure of the Lady is there to welcome you, to offer you congratulations and reward, recognition, and celebration, all things an infant requires for the healthy development of the first chakra. The Lady of the Lake is an important symbol in the legend of King Arthur, who reconnects to his destiny as symbolized by the sword Excalibur, which is found in the waters of the lake guarded by the Lady of the Lake. It is a centuries-old story of rebirth.

**The Native American sweatlodge** offers another variation on the Lady of the Lake, the advantage being this is something that can be undertaken with conscious effort, i.e., something that can be planned with the intention of bringing about this healing. You enter the lodge, i.e., the womb, where it is very dark. Prayers are offered by each person in the lodge. The heat inside the lodge is a purification that allows you and everyone else, at the end of the sweat, to emerge reborn, to offer one another congratulations and recognition.

**Rebirthing** is a technique whereby holotropic breathwork, a form of hyperventilation, is employed to access and purge traumatic early-childhood events that have been repressed.

**Quantum light breath** is a breathing meditation process that accelerates personal transformation by releasing withheld feelings and revealing unconscious programs. It combines elements of Vipassana meditation with deep rhythmic and consciously connected breath, to take a person into an expanded state of consciousness and ultimately into blissful embodiment of universal love, which is our natural state.

**Spiritual reconnection** to the person(s) directly connected to the source of your pain and missing energies in your first chakra. This is a reconnection to your mother or father in a state of meditation (a process covered in greater detail in chapter 3).

**Gold energy healing** uses gold energy, a form of subtle energy, to dissolve the black energy of pain from the body. You can find it inside yourself to heal yourself, or it can be channeled by someone else, such as a spiritual healer, into the parts of your body that require healing. Either way it can be used to heal the first chakra. The person requiring healing must, however, be willing to forgive the hurt that is causing their pain without knowing the particulars of the hurt. For example, if your father hurt you in your infancy, you must be willing to forgive your father for what he did, without knowing exactly what he did or why he did it. This is the way of gold energy healing. It forgives unreservedly.

**Self-welcome** is the practice of welcoming your inner child. At some point during the healing process of your first chakra you may feel the energetic presence of a little child, the "you" when you were in your mother's womb, release itself from deep within your lower abdomen, from a point midway along an imaginary line drawn between the rear of your navel and the space between L5 and SI in your spine. This energy point is known as the hara. When you feel her presence, say hello to her, give her recognition and welcome her. Allow her energy to radiate from that point into the rest of your body. Show her you love her. Show her that everyone in her family loves her, and tell her that you will always be there for her. You have to be, as you are her. This is the part of the journey where you heal your own first chakra.

## *The Second Chakra*

**Sanskrit name:** Svadhisthana
**Location:** Front, two finger widths below the navel; back, between L4 and L3
**Color:** Orange
**Element:** Water (yin/female, receiving, supportive)
**Vital functions:** Movement and the energy of movement; getting things done; the energy of life bursting forth, the source of physical energy; in massage and healing, the energy used to move the energy within the self and within another
**Symbols that appear in dreams and meditations:** Serpents, snakes, worms, and dragons; water in general; the sea, rivers and lakes (but not waterfalls, as in water falling from a source above, which represents the open sixth chakra and spiritual insight and intuition)
**Meridians:** Kidney; in yoga, the Ida and Pingala channels, or *nadis*
**Areas of the body:** Lower back, kidneys, adrenal glands, bladder; the sexual organs

### Developmental Needs

The second chakra relates to the things that drive young children from when a child first walks to about fourteen years of age, such as:

*Movement,* e.g., walking, running, dancing, playing in the playground, climbing, playing sports

*Curiosity,* e.g., when a child starts to grab everything within its reach or to put anything it can find into its mouth

*Sensation,* e.g., experiencing the five senses of taste, touch, smell, sight, and sound, as well as the ability to feel life in general

*Creativity,* e.g., drawing, painting, sculpting, music, playing dress up, performing, building things, and seeing the beauty in artistic expression

*Fun and playfulness,* especially involving others, e.g., smiling, laughter, happiness, silliness, joy, humor, playing games

*Innocence—spontaneous and immediate,* the way children easily make friends with other children; open to giving and receiving fully without judgment or expectation; yielding; doing things for the simple sake of doing things; not knowing why you do things, just doing them; playing games for the sake of playing, not to win, not for any reason, not corresponding to any rules

*Support and reassurance,* including the energy of support received by a growing child from her parents; if this energy is balanced and strong, it gives physical strength to the child in the areas of the lower back and knees; if it is weak or unbalanced, there will be parallel weakness in the lower back and knees. The energies of support and reassurance are very warming energies and can be used to counter the effects in the body of certain cold energies, most notably fear, fright, and shock. People with strong reserves of supportive energy are open and able to look after other people. They are not afraid of getting burned out from taking on the needs of others. The energies of support and reassurance are carried in the kidney meridian.

*Intimacy,* as in the way a parent holds the child fully when comforting or reassuring him following an accident or a fright. This type of touch is important in massage when bringing healing to a client who is holding the energies of shock or fright in the body.

## What the Energy of the Second Chakra Feels Like

As the energy of the second chakra is symbolized as water, it mirrors two aspects of water: it is cool, and it is heavy. Manifestations of second-chakra energy in the body include spongy skin, cool skin, cold skin, wet skin, sticky skin, contracted (tight) muscles; cold, dense, heavy muscles, for example, cold, dense, heavy, and contracted hamstring muscles; inflammation caused by a buildup of fluid; an area of the body that is very sensitive to being touched. When a large amount of second-chakra water energy is released into your body, it can make you hypersensitive to stimuli in your environment. It also makes you feel young, happy, and bright. It can make you laugh for no reason. It feels exciting and can lead to feelings of giddiness and silliness and wanting to have lots of fun, even such that you feel like you might lose control.

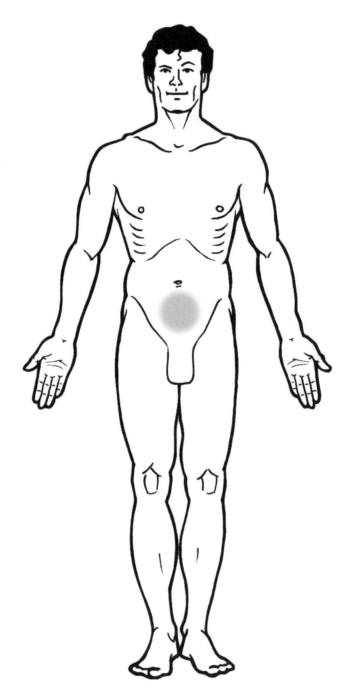

*Fig. 2.6. Location of the second chakra*

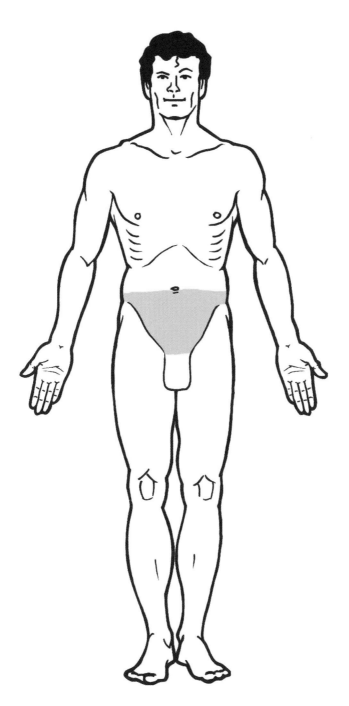

*Fig. 2.7. Area of the body governed by the second chakra (front)*

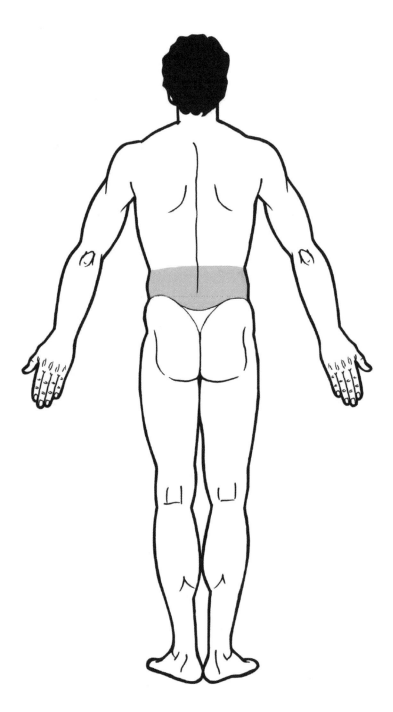

*Fig 2.8. Area of the body governed by the second chakra (back)*

The second chakra also houses the emotional energy of fear. The physical energy of fear has an enormously wide range of effects in the body. For instance, have you ever experienced heavy turbulence during a flight? If so, how did you feel? Dehydrated? Quiet? Nauseous? Introverted? Sweaty? Did your legs feel wobbly and did you have to go to the bathroom? Did your stomach tighten up and did your palms sweat? All these reactions are the result of a natural release of the emotional energy of fear from the second chakra.

When you focus a massage treatment on the second chakra, or on body areas associated with the second chakra, it is not unusual to feel any of these aforementioned reactions. Yoga asanas associated with the second chakra include cobra, boat, seated forward bend, supine bound angle, dog, cat, seated angle, balancing bear, and frog. A practice that focuses on these areas might also bring about any of the reactions listed above.

## Additional Functions

The second chakra also governs reproduction and sexual energy (sexual energy is explained in greater detail in chapter 4). It houses our feelings of lack and poverty and the feeling that there is not enough or that you do not have enough. The energy of the second chakra also has a smell, that of vomit.

### Using the Second Chakra in Massage

When students complete their first massage training and begin to practice on friends and family, their emphasis is usually on remembering sequencing and the use of correct technique within each subsequence. Students understandably remain in their head during this learning stage of their massage practice, and there is little or no awareness of subtle energy, and consequently no noticeable energy connection or energetic interplay between therapist and client. After some time, though, when you have the massage sequencing and technique down, you don't need to think about what to do next, you just know. During this stage, your focus moves from your head to your hands, from learning to touching. You begin to give yourself the space and time to feel what your hands are telling you about your client. This is a stage of curiosity, as you begin to inquire about the condition of your client and you begin to see whether what you learned in massage school can help alleviate the person's condition. This is the second stage in the development of one's massage practice: touching, sensing, and general curiosity, all second-chakra qualities. Therefore the first energetic connection with a client usually comes from the second chakra and extends through the sense of touch in the therapist's hands.

The use of your second-chakra energy in massage can sometimes stimulate second-chakra energy in your client. They are two separate energy centers of similar vibration, or frequency, which can begin to resonate with each other when brought into close contact. It is a natural occurrence, in the same way as when you run your finger along the rim of one of two similar wine glasses placed side by side, the other wine glass will spontaneously resonate along with the first glass. The challenging aspect of the second chakra is that it houses the energy of fear. Without any intention of doing so, you can inadvertently stimulate the energy of fear in your client with your massage. The double dilemma is that if you are not prepared for this, the stimulated energy of fear in your client can resonate with and stimulate the energy of fear in yourself. Although you may not experience the emotion of fear itself, you may experience the energy of fear in one of its more metaphysical forms: tiredness, heaviness, cold, nausea, or exhaustion. At this point many novice massage practitioners think they are taking on the "bad energy" of their client, but all that is happening is that the client's energy of fear is resonating with and stimulating the therapist's own hidden energy of fear. Although this can be uncomfortable and even frightening, it is not unusual when you are learning to work with energy in massage, and in time the effects will pass. You can, of course, use forms of protection to help you through this phase in your massage practice, such as visualizing a wall of gold between you and your client, visualizing yourself in a protective suit of armor, or placing yourself in a prana egg. Prayer is another extremely effective form of protection. The stronger the energy used in asking for protection through prayer and the stronger the prayers, the stronger the energy of protection experienced.

## The Third Chakra

**Sanskrit name:** Manipura
**Location:** Front, solar plexus; back, between L2 and L1
**Color:** Yellow
**Element:** Air (yang, male; the ability to destroy if untempered)*
**Vital functions:** The energy of conscious, mental activity; the center of the will
**Symbols that appear in dreams and meditations:** Sun, fire
**Meridians:** Stomach-spleen, liver-gallbladder
**Areas of the body:** Midback, digestive system, diaphragm, lower half of the chest cavity, stomach-spleen, liver-gallbladder

### Developmental Needs

The developmental needs of the third chakra relate to the period when a child is first able to reason till about twenty-one years of age. These needs govern one's abilities and understanding in the following aspects of life.

*Thought,* including reasoning, deduction, conscious understanding, decision-making, planning, direction in life, know-how, beliefs, and intellectually reasoned behavior

*Will,* i.e., the determination and ability to get things done, goal-setting, ambition, achievement, competition, and success

*Learning,* including all aspects of schooling and education; concentration, retention, and memory

*Law,* i.e., rules, rationale, and science

*Business,* including all aspects of business, money, and finance; financial success; advertising, marketing, and promotion

---

*There are differing opinions regarding the element governing the energy of the third chakra. Some authors describe the element as fire, while others say it is air. In my many years of teaching energy work wherein I allow students to discover the elements of the chakras through their own direct experience, no student has ever used the word *fire* to describe the energy of the third chakra, whereas *air, wind,* and *bubbles* are commonly mentioned. This experience supports my philosophy in teaching energy work to students, in which I allow students to discover the element of each chakra for themselves, without providing any information as to how it is described in books or by other teachers.

**Personal space,** including the setting up of personal space and
boundaries; shyness

**Attachment and ownership,** i.e., empire building, hierarchy, authority, control, unwillingness to let go, discipline, power-play

## What the Energy of the Third Chakra Feels Like

The energy of the third chakra is symbolized by the element of air,
which is neither heavy nor light, warm nor cool. Like air, however,
when third-chakra energy is released it creates pressure. Experiences of
third-chakra energy in the body include a buildup of air pressure, creating agitation, tension, and hardness across all bodily systems as well as
in the muscles and connective tissue. For example, third-chakra energy
is the energy that manifests as tight shoulders. Air pressure also leads
to headache and feelings of internal tightness, such as tightness across
the chest. An acute release of third-chakra air energy into the body can
also throw you off balance in the way strong windy weather does. It
is not uncommon to feel dizzy, lightheaded, slightly agitated, and not
quite yourself during a strong release of third-chakra energy into your
system. Third-chakra energy can also give rise to feelings of anger, rage,
frustration, impatience, revenge, intolerance, judgment, jealousy, unforgivingness, and violence.

By contrast, a strong release of third-chakra energy into the body
can also make you feel enormously confident, healthy, strong, and radi-
ant. A strong release of this energy into your body can stimulate your
mental functions and strengthen your will and determination to get
things done. It can also give you powerful feelings of achievement. The
feeling is as if you have a small sun shining from your solar plexus. A
massage client needing hard, pointed pressure in a treatment is usually
a person with a general excess of third-chakra energy throughout their
body.

When you focus on the third chakra in a yoga practice (including
bow, seated forward bend, upward boat, inclined plane, warrior I, warrior II, and half circle), or in a massage treatment, or focus on body
areas associated with the third chakra, it is not unusual to feel any of
the aforementioned sensations when this energy is released.

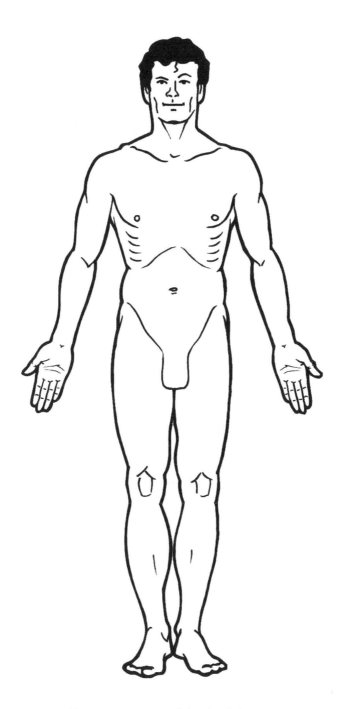

*Fig. 2.9. Location of the third chakra*

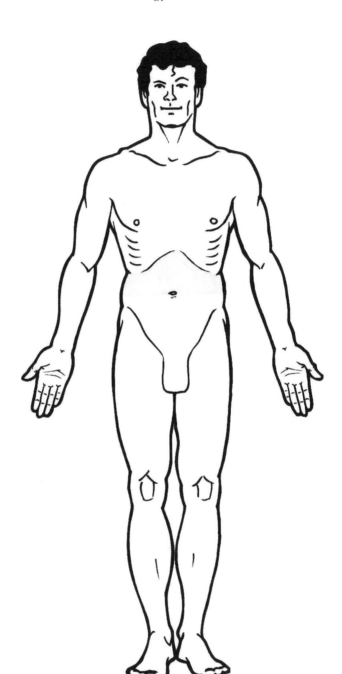

*Fig. 2.10. Area of the body governed by the third chakra (front)*

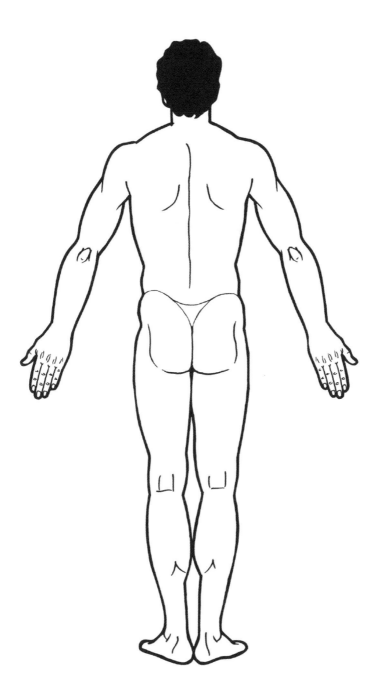

*Fig 2.11. Area of the body governed by the third chakra (back)*

## Additional Functions

The third chakra houses the energy we use in social situations, including our ability to socialize and make friends. It governs risk-taking, including betting and gambling. The energy of the third chakra also has a smell, that of when your mother used to use her spittle to clean your face when you were a kid.

---

### Using the Third Chakra in Massage

The next stage of development in the energy you use as your massage practice evolves and you gain more experience comes when you begin to see the results of your massage and you see that it works. You begin to realize you have the answers to certain disorders and can offer effective treatment. At this point your energy shifts from the second chakra, where you use your sense of touch to intuit what to do, back to the third chakra, where you first started out in massage school when you learned techniques, representing the third-chakra seat of learning and knowledge. This time, however, you do not stay in your head like when you first started practicing massage on friends and family. You now offer massage with the energy of knowledge that what you do works; it has been informed by the energy of the second chakra. This is a very strong and positive energy in massage, and if used with confidence and correct intention, it can bring about great results over the long term.

The use of third-chakra energy in massage can sometimes stimulate third-chakra energy in your client and, as before with the second chakra interplay, your client's stimulated third-chakra energy can resonate with your own. If a client's released third-chakra energy resonates with your third-chakra energy, you might experience feelings of agitation, anxiety, insecurity, frustration, impatience, or even anger. At this point, if you are not prepared for this, you might become insecure, frustrated, or impatient with your treatment or even angry at your client. This is understandable but misguided. What you are feeling and experiencing is nothing more than abstract third-chakra energy released by your client, which is now resonating with the energies housed in your own third chakra. If you ever feel agitated, dizzy, or suddenly lost or frustrated during a massage, pause a few moments, center yourself, and only then continue.

The feelings will dissipate. If you still experience any of these feelings post-massage, cut the energy connection between yourself and your client by visualizing a string, or energy meridian, running between you and your client that connects both of you at the third chakra, or solar plexus. Visualize grabbing hold of the string with one hand, and with two fingers of your other hand, make a scissors and cut the string. As a technique for cutting energy connections, this only works with new or very recent clients. Cutting the connection with longstanding clients requires the additional understanding of why your client needs the connection with you, and also why you allow the connection or why you also need the connection.

## The Fourth Chakra

**Sanskrit name:** Anahata

**Location:** Front, on the sternum, to the right of the heart; back, between the shoulder blades

**Color:** Green

**Element:** Fire

**Vital functions:** The giving and receiving of love in all its forms and the understanding of love in all its forms; the center of balance, the point where the energies of the lower chakras, one through three, are integrated with the energies of the higher chakras, five through seven

**Symbols that appear in dreams and meditations:** Flowers and fields of flowers; someone bringing you flowers (always note the person bringing the flowers); green fields and wide-open green spaces; treetops; someone bringing you something from your past that you once loved very much; a cathedral; an overflowing cup (e.g., the Holy Grail); a huge, dark, empty cave or room, revealing an open heart, but one that is empty of love

**Meridians:** Lung/large intestine; pericardium/triple heater; heart/small intestine

**Areas of the body:** The skin; heart, lungs, and upper chest; arms (outer upper arm, elbow joint, forearm, wrist, and hands); between the shoulder blades; shoulders (loneliness, sadness)

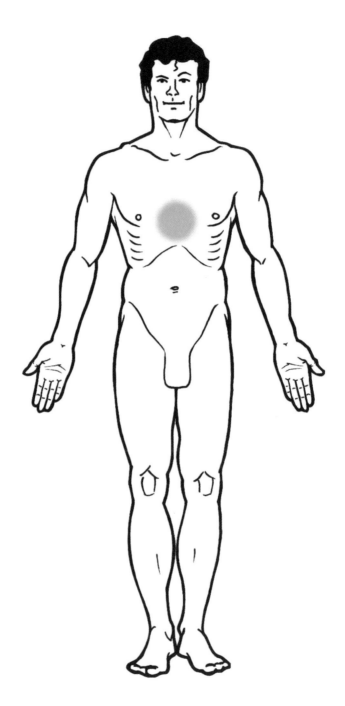

*Fig. 2.12. Location of the fourth chakra*

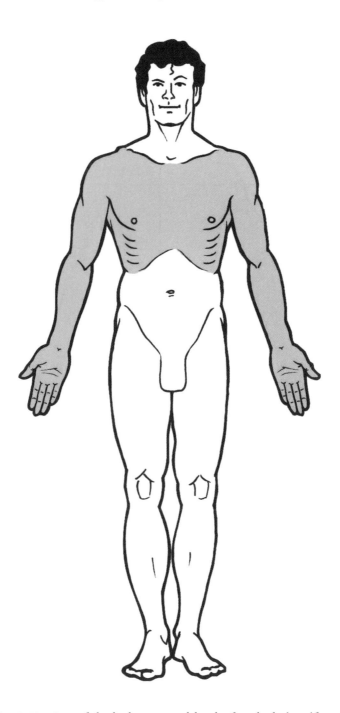

*Fig. 2.13. Area of the body governed by the fourth chakra (front)*

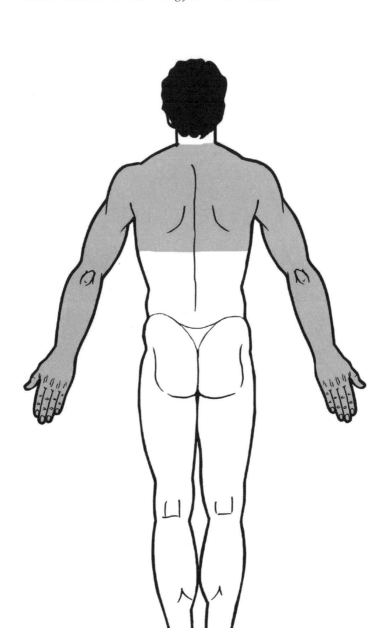

Fig 2.14. Area of the body governed by the fourth chakra (back)

## Developmental Needs

The developmental needs of the fourth chakra start at the period in life when you first fall in love and can last well into later life, depending on your experiences of being in love. The needs of the fourth chakra during this period of life include:

*Freedom,* the freedom to love without interference from any other chakra, such as the freedom to love another from the heart without the need for a sexual connection, a second chakra interference

*Equanimity,* the ability to see and treat everyone as equal

*Forgiveness,* including letting go and not being judgmental

*Life balance,* not the work-rest-play sense of balance, but the balance between family, feeling and enjoying the pleasures of life, intellectual activity, wealth, love, self-development, and spirituality

*Understanding,* the ability to see everything from both the rational, left brain, and spiritual, right brain, points of view

*Discernment,* the ability to differentiate between what is good for you and not good for you

Emotional energies damaging to the heart center are grief, sadness, loneliness, despair (loss of hope), and manic hysteria (e.g., the moment of excessive joy when you learn you have won the lottery). Mental, or behavioral, third-chakra energies that can damage the heart include unforgivingness, judging, not letting go, putting other people ahead of yourself or living your life through other people (i.e., relying on others for your own welfare).

## What the Energy of the Fourth Chakra Feels Like

A release of heart energy into the body can bring an overall sense of calm and space, as if you are sitting in a field of flowers in the wide open space of nature.

In yoga or massage, heart-centered energy can manifest as a welling-up of good feelings toward your students or clients, the spontaneous desire to hug your student or client, and the willingness to give without receiving in return. This feels like a complete openness and trust toward all aspects of life, and forgiveness of everyone. When you massage with fourth-chakra heart energy, you use an energy that transforms the energies of the greatest hurts and pains in your client's body. Massaging with strong fourth-chakra energy, there is no need for protection, as you cannot be hurt. When you focus a massage treatment or a yoga practice on the fourth chakra or on body areas associated with the fourth chakra, as in the yoga asanas fish, standing yoga mudra, pigeon, camel, standing backbend, and prayer twist, it is not unusual to feel any of the aforementioned reactions.

## Additional Functions

The fourth chakra is also regarded as the "great transformer," housing the energy that transforms darkness into light, pain into painlessness, tiredness into vitality, stress into calm, and struggle into freedom. The energy of the fourth chakra also has a smell, that of burning flesh.

## *The Fifth Chakra*

**Sanskrit name:** Visuddha

**Location:** Front, center front of the throat; back, center back of the neck

**Color:** Sky blue

**Element:** Ether

**Vital functions:** Truth; the ability to communicate clearly and truthfully; the ability to communicate your personal truth and your true beliefs, emotions, feelings, and needs, in the forms of speech, writing, or artistic creativity; the energy that can tell the difference between truth and illusion; the energy used in listening to intuit when someone is being untruthful to you

**Symbols that appear in dreams and meditations:** A wide-open skyscape; visions of people familiar to you, past or present, who represent the truth (e.g., a loving grandparent, the Buddha, Jesus, Leonardo da Vinci); fish (including whales and sharks); the Gospel story of Jesus feeding the crowd with loaves and fishes (i.e., feeding them with the nourishment of truth); dreams in which you are being strangled (usually the strangler is a male figure, representing the male ego trying to stop deep truth housed in the fifth chakra from being self-realized)

**Meridians:** The energy of the fifth chakra lies outside the realm of meridians; there are no meridians that carry fifth-chakra energy around the body

**Areas of the body:** Throat, mandible, and jaw muscles

## Developmental Needs

The governing need of the fifth chakra is the truth; the need for answers; the need for truthful answers. This need is triggered when someone is seeking the truth about a particular aspect of their life, such as *why hasn't my life worked out the way I hoped it would?* The fifth chakra is also triggered by the abstract feeling that some people in their late twenties or early thirties get that there is something missing in their lives. This is the fifth chakra calling the person to investigate some form of spiritual pursuit.

## What the Energy of the Fifth Chakra Feels Like

The effects of fifth-chakra energy in the body are very subtle. When released into the body, it can make you feel physically lighter or taller. It gives rise to feelings of mental and spiritual freedom, and your mind feels like it is expanding outward for miles and miles. Its energy has a very calming effect in the body. Gentle massage of the fifth chakra helps to release the muscles of the jaw and also melts tension in the upper half of the body. Yoga postures associated with the fifth chakra include fish, camel, standing backbend, half-shoulder stand, lion's face, and plow.

## Additional Functions

Fifth-chakra energy enables you to see beyond initial appearance to the underlying truth. This is incredibly useful in massage as it enables the therapist to see deeper into the ailment of the client. For instance if a client comes for massage complaining of shoulder pain, the therapist with a strongly

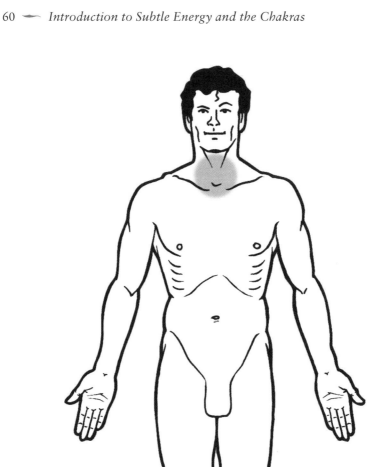

*Fig. 2.15. Location of the fifth chakra*

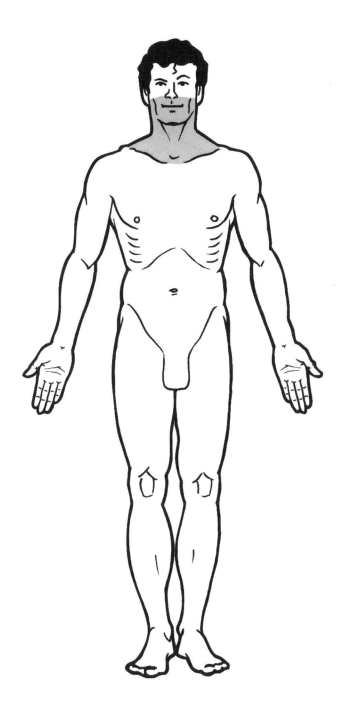

*Fig. 2.16. Area of the body governed by the fifth chakra (front)*

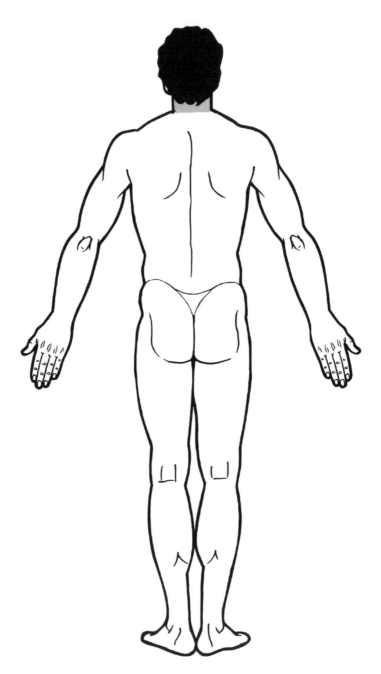

*Fig 2.17. Area of the body governed by the fifth chakra (back)*

functioning fifth chakra will be able to see deeper into the client's condition to the underlying cause of the shoulder pain, the truth of the matter.

## The Sixth Chakra

**Sanskrit name:** Ajna

**Location:** Front, center point between eyebrows (the third eye); back: center point at the back of the skull

**Color:** Indigo; also lilac or lavender, symbolizing deep awareness of the human condition; violet, a very powerful healing color; and deep, dark purple, an energy of an extraterrestrial source

**Element:** Light

**Vital functions:** Connection to the energies present outside our third-dimensional reality; connection to the energies of dead ancestors and family members; connection to the angel realm; the energy that transcends our references to location, time, and space; the energy that transcends all forms of duality and our ordinary beliefs regarding who we are and where we are; the feeling of merging into/with your environment; in massage, the energy to transcend the perceived physical boundaries separating therapist and client, leaving a feeling of the therapist and client being one; in yoga, a similar feeling of union between teacher and student; the turning upside down of commonly accepted beliefs about what is real and what is not; the truth is revealed in the opposite; heaven lies under your feet as well as above your head

**Symbols that appear in dreams and meditations:** People known to you who have passed on; your own self in past or future lifetimes or in life forms other than human, for example animal or plant; people you know appearing in alien form; water that descends from above (e.g., waterfalls); the Lady of the Lake, a symbol of rebirth; dreams and meditations in which a little girl appears to you (you do not recognize her face, but if you ask her who she is she will say she is you and is here to help and guide you)

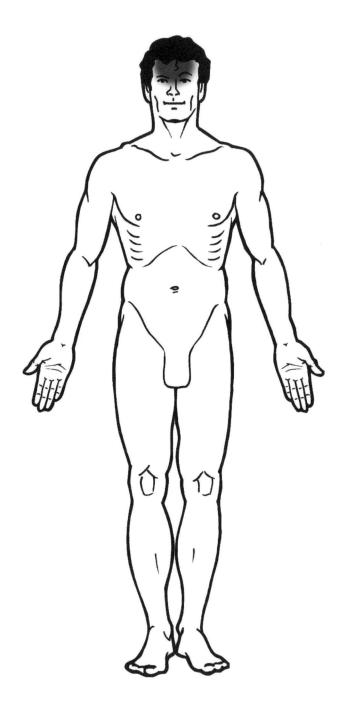

*Fig. 2.18. Location of the sixth chakra*

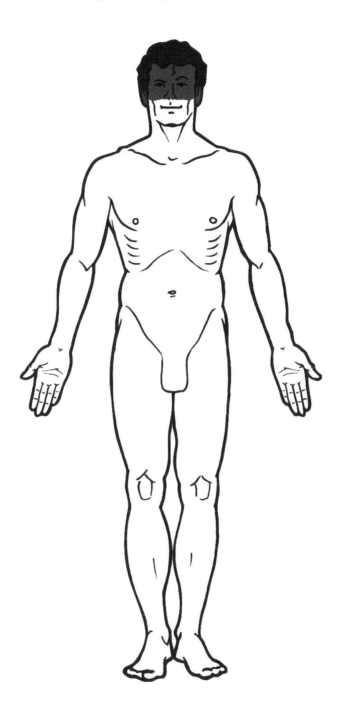

*Fig. 2.19. Area of the body governed by the sixth chakra (front)*

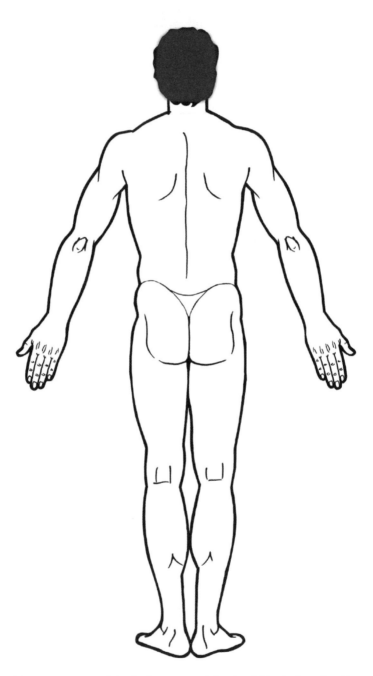

*Fig 2.20. Area of the body governed by the fifth chakra (back)*

**Meridians:** Similar to the fifth chakra, the energy of the sixth chakra lies outside the realm of meridians; there are no meridians that carry sixth-chakra energy around the body
**Areas of the body:** Forehead, back of head, temples, eyes, and ears

## Developmental Needs

The governing need of the sixth chakra, that of a spiritual understanding of life, is triggered by the needs of the fifth chakra. A person seeking the full truth behind a specific hurtful event in his life—for example, why he was abandoned by a parent—may need to use the energies of the sixth chakra to establish a higher-conscious connection to that parent. Through this he can uncover the forgotten, hidden, or unknown aspects of the parent's life, which are crucial in understanding why the parent acted a certain way.

## What the Energy of the Sixth Chakra Feels Like

The effects of the sixth chakra in the body are subtle. When this energy releases into the body it can make you feel like you are up in the clouds and very unattached to the ground beneath your feet. Metaphysically, the energy feels very hot; it is the hottest of all the subtle energies. Sixth-chakra energy strongly alters visual perception. It helps you to see the individual layers of gravity or the waves of energy that spread outward from your body as you exhale your breath. It helps you to see through the skin of people to their cellular level, like X-ray vision. It can give you the feeling of a sudden shift in your location within a three-dimensional space, where you do not physically move but your point-of-view perception of where you are shifts from your current location to a different location and then returns again, all within a split second (a form of bilocation). Sixth-chakra energy also gives rise to intuition and inspiration, making ideas come to you more quickly and more clearly. It helps you to see yourself more clearly in your future. Sixth-chakra energy also speeds up some of your normal functions. If you use sixth-chakra energy in massage, for instance, you will find that you need less time than normal to complete a successful treatment. Yoga asanas associated with the sixth chakra include child, seated head to knee, pyramid, side-seated angle, and meditation/shavasana.

## Additional Functions

The sixth chakra also houses the energy of spiritual love. Some people whose lives have been severely lacking in any form of earthly love, in particular familial love, seek and find the energy of spiritual love housed in the sixth chakra. This is often accomplished through meditation. The love of the sixth chakra is untainted by the human condition. It is a pure and clean love containing no pain, no judgment, and no bad memories. For many whose life is pain, the sixth chakra is the only place they feel free of pain.

---

### Using the Higher Chakras in Massage

Once you begin to gain experience and confidence in the use of energy in your massage practice, the next stage comes with the awakening of your own higher energy centers, i.e., the fifth and sixth chakras. How you awaken these energy centers, if indeed you even choose to awaken them, is your own choice. When I first studied Thai massage with Asokananda in the Lahu village, part of his teaching included early morning Vipassana meditation and, before class, chanting and prayer. Another great Thai massage teacher, Chaiyuth Priyasith, also prayed intensively to Lord Buddha, Shivago Komarpaj, and Kruba Srivichai before class, just as Pichest Boonthumme does. If you ever see the video about Thai massage that Asokananda plays at the start of his beginner's course, you will hear Pichest saying the reason why he meditates and prays is so he can "see." This does not refer to seeing with his eyes—it refers to a deeper form of seeing. This exemplifies the use of prayer and meditation to open your higher energy centers, energy that expresses itself as intuition or gut reaction.

As well as enabling you to see deeper into your client's condition, the use of higher-level energy in massage has certain metaphysical side effects. It can leave you feeling severely ungrounded or light-headed, and you can even lose touch with yourself and reality. It can leave you with a postmassage energy high, after which you then feel wiped out. It can also leave you feeling wonderfully happy, content, at peace with yourself, and spiritually fulfilled—which is why so many people desire this energy and often become addicted to finding it. If you ever experience any of these feelings postmassage, the best thing to do is to ground yourself deeply. Even though you may feel wonderful afterward, the feeling is meant to be temporary and not permanent. Do not become attached to it. When working with high energy in massage, you have to balance yourself by grounding deeply at the same time. If you do not ground yourself properly, continuous use of higher-level energy can cause severe imbalance in the mind.

The final stage in the evolution of the energy interplay between you and your clients comes one day when deep in the middle of a massage treatment you suddenly feel that there is no space or separation between you and the person you are massaging. The two of you have somehow become one, a sign that you are using the energy of your sixth chakra. In this stage, your concept of self-identity is altered, the physical boundaries that normally separate you from your client are no longer real, no longer tangible. The space in which both of you reside and in which the massage is taking place feels more like a huge soup of plasmalike energy without fixed form or boundaries. In the energy soup of your client, you find the energy of your own self already present.

When you find yourself in your client in this way, you will intuitively understand that your client cannot be anything else other than an extension of yourself, and that what you see or feel in your client is merely a reflection of what is already within you. There is no separation. There is no division. There is no other. There is only the oneness of an extended being. It is a moment of complete sixth-chakra spiritual clarity, and it is an incredibly liberating space to inhabit. Suddenly you are free and your massage is free.

## *The Seventh Chakra*

**Sanskrit name:** Sahasrara

**Location:** Outside the realm of the physical body, just above the crown of the head

**Color:** Purple. A growing presence of white occurs in a strongly opened seventh chakra

**Element:** Source, Atman, Tao

**Vital functions:** Freedom from mind, freedom from all forms of earthly experience: mental experience, emotional experience, and sense-based experience

**Symbols that appear in dreams and meditations:** A flash of incredibly bright white light, lasting only a fraction of a second, the brightness and power of the light shocks your energy body so strongly that it immediately awakens you and you feel afraid of it happening again, although you know the experience to be a good one. It is multiple times more powerful than kundalini energy. Subsequent visitations in dreams: the intensity of the white light diminishes, while the duration of the visits extend from a fraction of a second to a few seconds. When the intensity is sufficiently diminished, you are in the position to invite the light to enter your six bodily chakras. In reverse of the movement of the kundalini, white light energy descends downward through the chakras to the root. During some dreams, you are visited by a flash of forked lightning, which flashes downward through your chakras from the crown. This is a powerful electricity-like feeling that jolts you awake. The more strongly your chakras are open, the deeper the lightning strikes into you.

### Developmental Needs

The seventh chakra neither recognizes nor understands the concept of need, as need is a conscious mind construct. It has no needs.

### What the Energy of the Seventh Chakra Feels Like

The seventh chakra is a state of being. Not of the body, it cannot be described using the words of the body, such as sense-based

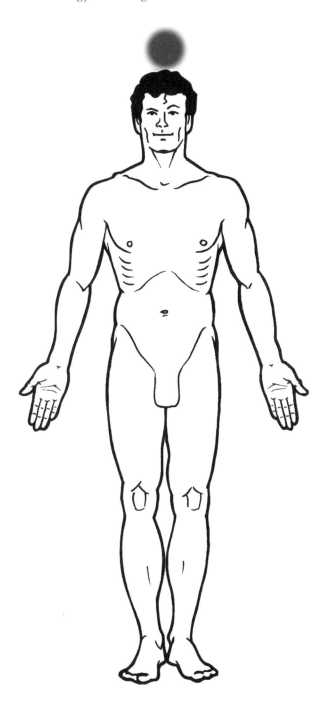

*Fig. 2.21. Location of the seventh chakra*

descriptions. It does, however, have the appearance of white light. No emotional or mental process takes place in this state of being. This state of being does not understand the language and experiences of the body. It does not understand our experience on Earth. There is no thought or thinking present in this state. There is no communication with the light. And this is its joy. There is no communication because there is no judgment, and in that moment of realization, there is total, absolute freedom. Freedom from all aspects of mind. In the state of seventh chakra white light, there is no sense of any other being. No other. Only self.

## Sensitivity to Energy in Massage

Each of us has a unique natural energy level that differs from any other person. Some people are naturally sporty, others naturally good with money, while others make great parents. Sports, finance, and parenting—examples of the myriad of energy possibilities—use very different energies. If you are naturally good at one, it indicates you have a natural energy for it.

In massage, it is extremely helpful to know your natural energy level. I say this for two reasons. First, it can guide you in a direction that is best suited to you in your massage practice. For instance, is your energy better suited to the use of massage as a physical therapy; massage as a pleasurable, relaxing, or sensual experience; as a medical treatment; as compassionate work; or as spiritual healing? This is very important to know because if you try to offer a style of massage that requires a level of energy that is outside your natural level, you will find that your work tends to make you tired. If you try to work at the level of the heart, offering loving and compassionate work, when your natural energy is at the level of the solar plexus, which houses the natural energy for medical diagnosis and treatment, it will slowly make you more and more tired. This is not to say you cannot work at the level of the heart if your heart is not your natural energy level, but it is to say that to do so will cause you to use more energy than you normally use in your nonmassage environment.

The same principle applies if you are a yoga teacher who is maybe trying to teach your yoga in a style, or energy, that lies outside your natural energy level.

To discern your natural energy level, you can use the services of a good energy worker, spiritual healer, or clairvoyant. This is quite easy to do. I did this with my teacher Jasmine Vishnu in Chiang Mai. We discovered that the energy I naturally use in my massage work is blue green in color. With reference to the chakras and the colors of the chakras, blue green refers to a frequency, or vibration of energy, that lies between the frequencies of the fourth chakra, a green energy, and the fifth chakra, a sky blue energy.

## Chakra Imbalances

Chakra imbalances may be of three types: empty, depleted, and excessive. If a chakra has been starved of much of its environmental energetic needs during its stage of development, it is said to be empty. For instance, a child born into an austere environment, starved of the energies of love, support, fun, and playfulness, will end up with a first chakra almost devoid of the energies needed for its healthy development. Not only will the first chakra be said to be empty, but the energy meridian charged with carrying the energy of the first chakra around the body, the urinary bladder meridian, will similarly be said to be empty of energy, or in TCM terms *chi* (or *qi*).

A chakra becomes depleted when its store of energy is overused. This applies mostly to the second and third chakras. The second chakra, among other things, stores the energy we use to move and get things done—it stores physical energy. When we physically overwork, the energy of the second chakra becomes depleted, and this is mirrored in a weakened condition of the body areas and organs associated with the second chakra: the lower back and the kidneys. Restoring energy to a depleted chakra is relatively easy and usually involves rest and proper nutrition. TCM treatment is highly effective in restoring depleted energies to the chakras and meridians.

If a chakra has been overfed with environmental energies during its stage of development, that chakra is said to be excessive. For instance, a child born into an environment lacking in love and play may be extremely well provided for both financially and educationally. The child may be provided with all the possessions he desires, given plenty of money, and may also be provided with extremely high levels of education and career help. These are all the energies of the third chakra. As a result of this kind of overnutrition, the third chakra may be said to be in an imbalanced state of excess, and the channels charged with carrying third-chakra energy around the body—the stomach, spleen, liver, and gallbladder meridians—may also be described as being in an imbalanced state of excess.

A chakra also becomes excessive when it is unable to dissipate energy into the adjacent chakras, i.e., those above and below it. This condition mostly applies to the second, third, and fourth chakras. It is not unusual to find practitioners of the more dynamic forms of yoga using their practice to dissipate the energy of their third chakra through their practice, as they are unable to ground this energy downward through their root chakra, legs, and feet, or upward through their heart chakra. This may be because the first chakra is empty, which is then mirrored in a state of semiemptiness in the fourth chakra, which is paired with the first chakra. When a chakra is empty, energy is unable to flow freely through it and through the meridians running through it. A rough metaphor for this can be seen when you suck the air out of a drinking straw and then hold the straw at both ends. The straw, as a metaphor for an energy channel, or meridian, is said to be empty of air, or empty of energy. In this state it is unable to allow anything to flow through it.

## Chakra Imbalance as a Comfort Zone

It almost goes without saying that just about everyone on Earth is in a state of energy imbalance. We are either born this way, i.e., as a result of nature, or have become this way, i.e., as a factor of nurture. Children born into families where there has been a strong history of control or of not showing emotion running through the

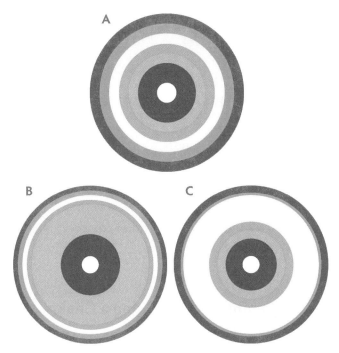

*Fig 2.22. Representations of three chakra types:*
*(a) balanced chakra; (b) imbalanced chakra with excess of blue and indigo and*
*lack of red, orange, yellow, and green, which reveals a person who has sought*
*solace in spiritual pursuits, such as meditation and prayer, in an attempt to*
*get away from life; (c) imbalanced chakra with excess of yellow and lack*
*of red and orange, which reveals a person who has been well*
*provided for educationally, financially, and professionally,*
*but their life is lacking in familial love, fun, and play*

generations will be born with an imbalance in their first chakra, an excess in the third layer, and blockages in the second and fourth layers. Children brought up in a cold, unloving home environment will develop an imbalanced first chakra as well as an imbalance in the red and orange layers in all of their other chakras. The energy imbalance in the first chakra is caused by a lack of or even an absence of certain energies normally belongiong to the first chakra, specifically the loving, playful, and supportive energies necessary in childhood. In contrast, children brought up in an environment where they are given everything they need in terms of money, possessions, education, career help, and guidance, and who are told they can achieve anything they want, will form an imbalance in their third chakra; the imbalance is caused by an excess of yellow, air energy, and will be mirrored by a similar layer of excess yellow energy in all the other chakras.

Whether due to nature or nurture, any child growing into adulthood will become so accustomed to their state of energy imbalance that it feels normal, even natural to them. They *feel* like they are balanced because the way they are today is the way they have always been. The imbalanced state has become a kind of comfort zone that defines what it feels like to be "me."

## Opening and Balancing a Chakra

To balance a chakra, there needs to be energy freely running through all the aspects of your life that are represented by the different colors of the chakras, to make for a little bit of everything in life. Accordingly, you need to establish a balance within all the different layers of energy within the chakra, as seen in figure 2.2 on page 28, from the energies of family/red energy, all the way out to the energy of spirit/purple energy, such that there is an equal amount of energy running through each of the seven layers, or colors, of the chakra. This takes time. It is not something achievable in a weekend workshop.

One of the first things that happens when you open and vitalize a chakra is that the new and sudden movement of powerful energy within your body causes you to experience your spatial relationship with your environment to be shaken in a left-right direction that can sometimes feel unpleasant, almost like travel sickness or vertigo. Your environment is not actually moving, of course, but your perception of it is. This is your energy affecting your perception of what you see with your eyes. This is one of the ways the energy of a chakra reveals its presence—it alters your perception. One of the other ways chakra energy can alter your perception is that it can make you feel like you are seeing things.

This could be a color, an image, or a symbol that you see in your mind's eye, or a vivid memory of something in your past. Sometimes chakra energy alters what you see in your dreams, especially the energy found in the higher chakras in the body.

Once you have begun to vitalize and open a chakra, the experience of left-right shaking in your spatial relationship turns into an elliptical movement, which soon after turns into a circular movement. The feeling of circular movement reflects the circular movement of energy within the chakra you are opening, indicating that the chakra is now open and ready for the process of healing or balancing. It may take from two or three hours to two or three days for this process to complete, depending on how intensely you work and how much time you have to work. An important caveat here is never attempt to open your own chakras yourself; always use the services of an appropriately trained guide, teacher, or energy worker.

When a chakra is balanced, the new state of balance unlocks a

*Fig. 2.23. The movement of energy within a chakra as it opens, from top to bottom: still, left-right, elliptical, and circular*

previously hidden form of energy from within the chakra. It is as if your chakra sends you a message letting you know it is balanced. This message is perceived as a symbol that you can clearly see in your mind's eye. You cannot miss this symbol—it has a very large presence in your mind. There is a specific symbol that means "chakra balanced," and only when you see this symbol in your imagination do you know that the specific chakra you have been working on is now balanced. It is the same symbol for all chakras. A genuine teacher or expert practitioner who has balanced his or her own chakras will know what this symbol is and so will be able to guide you to this symbol.

Chakra balancing should not be judged on a feel-good basis. If a teacher or guide tries to convince you your chakras are balanced on the sole basis that you feel good, you are being misinformed.

## Balancing All the Chakras

When all your chakras are balanced, this state of balance releases another specific symbol into your imagination. Teachers who have worked on themselves sufficiently to balance all their chakras will know what this symbol is and will be able to guide you to this symbol too. It is different from the symbol that signifies the achievement of balance in a single chakra.

Another way to know you have balanced all your chakras is when you have a dream in which you are asked to integrate twelve types of energy. The twelve energies are divided into six pairs, with each pair representing yin and yang aspects. The six pairs of polar energies you are asked to integrate are:

1. Yin and yang (symbolizing your own internal female and male energies)
2. Mother and father (i.e., your parents)
3. Young and old
4. Up and down
5. Black and white
6. Known and unknown (i.e., intellect and intuition)

When you know how to integrate or balance these six pairs of energies, you are said to have learned the lessons of your earth body's six chakras; this means that the chakras of your higher body, the seventh chakra and the higher minor chakras, are now opened to you.

## Balancing the Energy of a Meridian*

There is a close relationship between the chakras and the meridians. A chakra is like a geographical region in a country, while a meridian is a river running through that region. In your body, a chakra is a specific region or area where a specific type of energy is found. For example, in your fourth chakra you will find the energy of your heart. The rivers, or meridians, running through your heart chakra transport the energy of your heart wherever they flow. This is why sometimes when you are working to open or vitalize a chakra you will additionally vitalize or energize any meridian running through that chakra.

If you work to energize a specific point on a meridian, known in TCM as an acupuncture point, it can feel like a short, sharp pinprick, tingling, or pain. If you energize a section of a meridian it can feel like a zing of electricity running between two points inside you. The sensations of a meridian opening are different from the sensations of a chakra opening. Although in both cases the sensations are manifestations of energy, the way the energy of your chakras speaks to you is different than the way the energy of your meridians speaks to you. The same applies to the way a chakra reveals its state of balance to you and the way a meridian reveals its state of balance to you: they are each different.

A chakra reveals a state of balance by sending you a message in the form of a symbol, which you clearly see in your mind's eye, as previously mentioned. A meridian reveals its state of balance by sending you a different symbol, in the form of a combination of two colors, which you will also clearly see in your imagination. A teacher or guide who has balanced the energies in his or her own meridians will know what this

---

*In addressing this subject I am referencing the system of energy meridians as defined by Traditional Chinese Medicine (TCM).

color combination is and so will be able to guide you to find this color combination too.

It should be noted that once a state of energy balance in a chakra or meridian is established, this is not a permanent state. A state of balance is almost always transitional. In terms of personal development, the point in achieving a state of balance, whether in a chakra or in a meridian, is to learn the life lesson contained in the energy of that particular chakra or meridian. Once you have learned and understood the lesson it is let go, and the corresponding chakra or meridian is set free. In its newfound state of freedom, the need for that chakra or meridian to be balanced no longer applies and you are now free to move on to the next chakra or meridian that needs balancing.

# Balancing Yin and Yang

Of all the systematic classifications of subtle energy that can be balanced, the duality of female and male, yin and yang, is probably the most important. The benefits of being female-male-energy balanced are incredibly important in massage, especially if, as a massage therapist, your intention is to bring healing. If, as a massage therapist, you are not female-male balanced within yourself, you will not be able to sense the balance and quality of your client's internal female and male energies. Similarly, if you are a yoga teacher, you will only be able to help your students achieve the all-important balance of female energy, as seen in postures for promoting growth, clearing energetic blockages, and enhancing circulation, and male energy, as seen in postures that develop core strength and muscle tone, balance, and stamina, if you yourself have acquired some level of yin-yang balance within your own practice.

The bottom line is that as long as you remain in a state of energy imbalance in your own body, you will not be able to discern a state of imbalance in the body of another person. Nor will you be able to discern balance. In other words, to be able to discern imbalance you first have to be able to differentiate between balance and imbalance, and you cannot do this if you have never balanced yourself.

## Discovering Your Yin-Yang, Female-Male Energy

It's essential in massage, and quite helpful in yoga, to discover the balance of our internal yin-yang, female-male energy so that we can be effective in working with clients and students and bring deeper insight into our own practice. Most of us have an imbalance between our internal male and female energies. Some of us are said to be more male, while some of us are said to be more female. Find out which. If you find you have a greater percentage of male than female energy, it means your energy is more suited to working with male energy (men, in general) than female energy (women, in general). Working with male energy won't tire you out as much as working with female energy. The tiredness may not be noticeable in the early stages of your massage career, but over time the amount of tiredness in you can subtly build to a chronic level. If you don't already know it, you can discover the balance of your internal male and female energies by consulting with an energy worker, spiritual healer, or clairvoyant. It is relatively easy to find out.

Let's say, for example, you are a male massage therapist working with a female client. If in your own life your father was the dominant force in your parent's relationship, then a copy of that male-dominant energy was passed on to you at the time of your conception and you therefore carry an internal male-dominant energy in your own body. Now let's say that one of your client's great pains is that she has always been under the control of a domineering male figure, initially her father, and then subsequently her partners and spouse. Now she comes to you seeking help, or healing. If you, as her healer, are not internally female-male balanced, you will not be able to sense that the female energy in your client has been hurt by a domineering male energy, and you will embark on healing her in massage using your own internal male-dominant energy. This will only serve to reinforce your client's position and will not heal her of her pain. The great paradox in such a massage is that your client may actually feel good after your treatment, but all that has happened is that you have reinforced the imbalance already present in her. For your client, her life of imbalance is the only sense of "balance" she has ever had, i.e., in her state of imbalance she feels balanced. Your massage reinforced this imbalance; hence she feels balanced. You think you've done a great job. Have you?

If you are a male therapist with an internal male-dominant energy, you have two choices in this situation: you can massage her using only your female energy, or you can massage her with your female energy being supported by your male energy. The latter is the more healing energy to use, but initially it will be difficult for your client to trust it and open to it, as she has been hurt, and not supported, by male energy for so long. She will respond more easily to you when you use only your female energy.

There are various techniques for massaging a person with either female or male energy, or with a mixture of male-supporting-female energy or female-supporting-male energy. You will discover these techniques yourself through your own self-development in your massage practice. If I were to detail these techniques here, there is a danger they will be copied and used without proper understanding, and this would only cause further hurt.

As a massage therapist, the way you know you are internally female-male balanced is when you first touch a client with both your hands, you intuitively sense which hand your client is more open to receiving from.

## Left Side, Right Side of the Body

In general, the left-hand side of the body is said to be the yin, female side of the body. The energy connections between you and your mother and between your mother and her family are to be found on the left side of the pelvic girdle and the left upper leg and left lower leg. Customarily, the right-hand side of the body is said to be the yang, male side. The energy conections between you and your father and between your father and his family are to be found on the right side of the pelvic girdle and right upper leg and right lower leg. However, there are instances in which this polarity is sometimes reversed.

Indeed, the yin-yang, left-side/right-side polarity of any energy center, or chakra, in the body can be reversed. There is no precise explanation for why this happens—some people are simply polarity-reversed.

In addition, your mother is born of both the male and female energies of her parents, and if this energy strongly favors male energy, then the balance of yin-yang, female-male energy housed in your left leg can actually be male. Similarly, your father is born of both male and female energy, and if this energy strongly favors female energy, then the balance of yin-yang, female-male energy within your right leg can actually be female. Add to this the fact that there is also a tendency for energy from the lower left side of the body to cross over to the upper right side of the body at the point of the navel, and for the energy from the lower right side of the body to cross over to the upper left side of the body.

Because of these contradictions within the generally held belief of left-side female energy, right-side male energy, when it comes to energy balancing in massage, it makes no difference whether you start on the left or right side of the client's body.

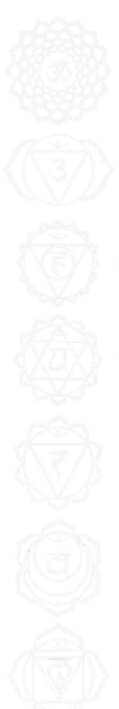

# PART TWO

# Types of Subtle Energy and Their Release through Yoga and Massage

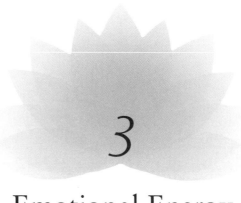

# 3

# Emotional Energy

Emotional energy is much more than the experience of an emotion itself; it is also that which fuels and gives rise to the emotion. Before the actual experience or outburst of emotion, the energy that gives it form builds up in your body, and as it does so it affects your body in a wide range of physiological and metaphysical ways. Some emotional energies have a warming, expansive, and strengthening effect on the body; others have an agitating, hardening effect; and still others have a cooling, contracting, weakening effect. These characteristics can be found not only in the muscles and connective tissues in the body, but across all systems of the body: respiratory, digestive, nervous, muscular, skeletal, endocrine, circulatory, lymphatic, urinary, and reproductive.

## Eight Emotional Energies

The following describes the physiological and metaphysical character-istics and effects of eight of the most commonly experienced emotions and feelings. It is hoped that by sharing this information, you will be able to better understand your own body as well as be better able to help others who experience the same effects of the emotions.

## Fear

All emotions have some degree of physiological or metaphysical effect on the body, but two emotional energies, fear and anger, have the widest range of noticeable effects. And of all the emotional energies, the physiological effects of the energy of fear can be the most difficult to understand, simply because one of the first reactions we have to fear energy being released in the body—for example, during a yoga practice or massage treatment—is to try and stop it. It is not unusual during a massage for a client experiencing the rising signs of fear to say, "Stop, this is making me feel uncomfortable," or "I don't like what is happening," or "I don't want to go any further."

Most people ordinarily do not voluntarily investigate the energy of fear, and because of this they do not understand the adverse effects the hidden or unconscious energy of fear has on the body. Notably, some of the fear energy stored in your body today can relate to issues and events originating deep in your past, and these events are probably forgotten or buried. But just because you have forgotten the fearful events from your past does not mean that the energy relating to those events is no longer stored in your body. The body can hold on to the energy of fear for a long, long time, even though the conscious mind may have forgotten or blocked out the event that triggered the original fear.

The lack of conscious awareness of the effects of fear energy can lead to many misunderstandings and misinterpretations of certain physical symptoms that may present in the body, such as chronic, low-level nausea, coldness in the abdomen, weakness in the lower back, tiredness, heaviness, tight hamstrings, closed hips, etc. Misinterpreting the true source of such physical problems can then lead to inappropriate and/ or ineffective courses of treatment, many of which serve only to further bury the hidden emotional energy at the root of the problem, or even worse, cause additional and completely unnecessary harm.

It is not uncommon to experience the energy of fear, although in a milder form, if you are practicing a series of yoga asanas designed to stimulate the second chakra (e.g., cobra, boat, seated forward bend, supine bound angle, dog, cat, seated angle, balancing bear, and frog), or while giving or receiving an intense massage that inadvertently releases second-chakra energy. You may not feel the emotion of fear as you have come to know it outright in its more obvious forms, as described in the discussion of the second chakra in chapter 2, but you may well experience one or more of its less recognized physiological and/or metaphysical side effects:

- An overall feeling of coldness or a release of coldness from deep inside a part of your body
- Cold sweats
- Shivering, low-level internal shaking, chicken skin, goosebumps, or hair standing on end
- A change in the rhythm of breathing, from full and relaxed to shallow and contracted
- A sudden feeling of tiredness, exhaustion, or a feeling of having no energy
- An overall feeling of heaviness, especially heaviness in the legs
- Legs can feel very cold or numb, especially in the backs of the legs, or can also sometimes feel cold and wobbly, like cold jelly
- Dehydration or dry lips
- A complete loss of appetite
- The inability to talk to anyone; not enough energy for conversation
- The inability to look someone else in the eye; insufficient energy to hold the gaze of another person
- A dull or intense feeling of nausea, sometimes leading to vomiting
- Diarrhea (too much cold energy in the large intestine)
- A greater-than-normal need to pee (a sign of the kidneys detoxifying)
- Extreme sensitivity to touch or being touched
- Loss of color in the complexion; going pale or white

When during the course of a massage or yoga practice any of these experiences of fear energy are triggered, it may be inconvenient or even uncomfortable, but this kind of release is normal and natural and should pass within a short while, or at most within two to three days. If the symptoms persist, however, it may reveal the remaining energetic presence of an event in your life that once caused you to be terribly afraid and is still causing you to feel the energy of fear in the present.

If you are more sensitive to energy, you may additionally experience an abstract feeling of blackness or stickiness within yourself. In your dreams at night you may see pictures of thick, black motor oil or black witches or black, fearful-looking creatures. And if you are able to sense the colors of energy, you will sense the color black when you touch the energy of fear in someone. These physiological and metaphysical experiences reveal the presence of the energy of fear in your own or another person's body. The level of energy is not yet strong enough to trigger the actual emotion of fear itself, nor is it strong enough to reveal the event that caused the original fear. Yet it is possible in a strong yoga or massage practice to intentionally raise the level of fear energy in your body such that you can reveal and release its underlying origin.

## A Conversation with Fear

Fear has been the major emotional issue in my life, stemming all the way back to my life in the womb. I have had to confront my fear on multiple occasions during the first thirteen years of my self-development, which I started in 2002 at age forty. On one such occasion, in August 2009, the blackness of fear came to me one night, and from a dream in which I was sitting in darkness on the sandy floor of a pyramid it woke me and spoke to me. I was able to write down what it told me.

"We [Fear, which is both female and male] are only a power, a force. We cannot harm you. Nothing can harm you. We are the darkness all around you. These great stone statues you touch in the darkness are your own great, untouched potential. [The statues were present in the dream in the base of the pyramid.] The darkness is all around, but the light is within, so breathe in the darkness. You chose the female form for us. You enter the darkness through the vagina. [Fear of women was the dominant form of fear in the male side of my family, going back three generations. Each of us has our own individual symbol, or chosen form, for fear.] The darkness slows you down, makes you afraid, makes you cold. Your hands get wet, the sand [in the dream] sticks to them. After a while you can crawl no more [in the blackness on the floor of the pyramid]. You bow your head down, afraid of what you might see in the complete darkness. Voices and whispers fly all around you. You are lost. You don't know where you are. You don't know what is in front of you. You don't stop moving completely, because you know that to do so would mean death. So you keep moving forward. Very slowly. But you also begin to realize that nothing bad has happened yet. Although you are surrounded by darkness and fear, you are still untouched, unharmed. We cannot hurt or harm you. We are inert power and force. All we do is slow you down and stop you from discovering the truth. It is fear that makes you feel alone and believe in loneliness. It is not being alone or lonely that makes you afraid. Fear precedes loneliness. Loneliness is born out of fear. And although fear is a darkness that terrifies you, you can talk to it. You can talk to fear. You can ask it questions. You can ask who it is. And it will answer. And it will teach you. It is open and willing to do this. Fear will teach you, if you only let it. And it is quite gentle in its replies. It doesn't even shout or roar. In its own way fear wants you to breathe it in. By doing so, it is mixed with the light within and is set free. Your reward is then your own potential."

## What the Energy of Fear Feels Like in the Body of a Massage Client

If you are a massage therapist and you like to start a treatment at your client's feet, check to see if the feet feel cold and hard and if the skin is wet or sticky. If you are unsure about what you feel at the feet, move to the calves and check to see if they too are cold, hard, wet, or sticky. Cold, hard, moist skin is indicative of the presence of the energy of fear in the body area you are treating. If the skin is sticky, it indicates a stronger presence of the energy of fear, as stickiness is a quality of fear energy. There is no scientific proof of this, but when you spend a few years treating clients who hold excessive amounts of fear energy in their bodies, you will have felt all the proof you need.

Be mindful when treating a client presenting with such symptoms, as the person may be carrying buried fears and memories relating to an event in her past, an event she may not wish to revisit at this time. The effect of your massage could disturb these old energies and bring to the surface memories of the event. If you see this happening, ask the person if she feels comfortable enough to continue the massage. If not, you may have to pause until she regains sufficient comfort to allow you continue the massage. If she is unable to regain sufficient comfort, you may have to stop the massage completely. If, on the other hand, she wants you to continue, you may end up guiding her through deeper and deeper layers of emotional energy as they become revealed, and then released, through the massage.

## Anger

The energy of anger can pervade the body, with a wide range of adverse effects across all bodily systems. It is, however, not quite as uncomfortable or as difficult to deal with and release as fear is.

There are two types of anger: simple anger and complex anger. Simple anger is an expression of anger related to a single event—for example, the anger at having a bad toothache or a pounding headache. Complex anger is an expression of anger related to a series of events, such as anger at work or anger at life. Complex anger is an umbrella emotion made up of parts of other energies, such as frustration, impatience, jealousy, hatred, bitterness (anger and sadness mixed together), disappointment, unforgivingness, intolerance, judgment, the need to punish, the need for revenge, the feeling of injustice, the feeling of being controlled, the experience of having your personal power undermined or taken away, and the feeling of loss, such as a job loss and the subsequent feeling of entitlement following such a loss or injustice. Rage is an expression of complex anger allowed to explode.

I have grouped these feelings, experiences, beliefs, and behaviors together because the energies that fuel and give rise to them have a common origin or starting point within the body. This starting point is the third chakra, located in the solar plexus (refer to chapter 2 for a detailed description). Due to their common energy and origin, all these particular emotions, feelings, experiences, and behaviors have similar physiological and metaphysical effects on the body.

An easy way to describe the physiological effects of the energy of anger is to list some examples of common situations where this energy is released into the body. If you can relate to any of these examples, reflect on how you felt at the time and how your body felt too.

- Waiting in a long line in the supermarket to pay for a few groceries while at the top of the line an elderly person dithers for ages trying to get the right amount of money out of her purse, and then begins to count out exact change
- Fighting to be first to get on a full train or bus during evening rush hour, then just as you are about to successfully board, being pushed aside by someone else trying even harder than you to get on the same train or bus
- Being stuck in traffic when you need to get to the airport quickly in order to catch your flight
- Finding that you have locked yourself out of your car or apartment
- Trying to get to sleep the night before an important exam or job interview
- Having your car stolen, clamped, or ticketed
- Having someone beat you in a sporting event, game, or test of intelligence you wanted to win
- Having only $100 left in your bank account when there is still two weeks to go till your next paycheck
- Being given a mundane task to do by your employer who knows you hate doing that job and who also knows there is nothing you can do about it
- Living through a week of very strong windy weather

Such a list could go on forever, but what you begin to see is that the effects of all these different scenarios in the body are basically the same:

- You feel agitated
- You feel tense
- You have a hard time remaining calm or still
- You are not able to ground yourself through your legs and feet
- You may find you are unable to concentrate, remember, or even think
- Your breathing moves to your upper chest and becomes shallower
- You feel a need to vent or you may explode
- Clenching in some part of your body
- Losing some, but not all, of your appetite
- Some foods and beverages make you feel ill
- Disturbed sleep

From this list there are three key characteristics to understanding how anger energy, or energy from the third chakra, feels in your body: 1) it makes parts of your body and certain muscles harden, the most common areas being the midback, shoulders, and jaws; 2) you cannot fully connect to yourself or somehow do not feel quite right in your own skin, or you are unable to ground yourself; and 3) you lose your natural ability to digest a full range of foods and beverages because they make you feel nauseous. When you experience any of these feelings during or after a strong massage session, it shows that there has been a release of anger-type energy from your third chakra into your system. This is a natural occurrence and should be no cause for alarm. Be aware too that if in yoga you follow a set of asanas designed to open the third chakra (e.g., bow, seated forward bend, upward boat, inclined plane, warrior I, warrior II, and half circle), you might experience sensations as a result of your practice. They are all natural to the third chakra, as are the positive aspects and feelings of an open third chakra, such as any feelings of success, achievement, and added confidence.

If, however, the uncomfortable feelings and sensations persist, it reveals a chronic excess of anger-type energy or a strong imbalance of third-chakra energy in your body. This is your body calling on you to investigate these feelings and sensations more deeply until their cause or origin is revealed. When the origin is fully revealed, then the energy of the event can be released and the body set free of the physiological and metaphysical manifestations caused by the energy. This is the journey of healing through energy work.

## Jealousy

Many people say they are not prone to jealousy, but there is a type of jealousy the energy of which you may be carrying in your body, but which you may be totally unaware of, and that is the jealousy that another person has of you.

There can be people in your life who are secretly jealous of you. They can be secretly jealous of the amount of sexual attention you receive from people. They can be jealous of your success at work or in education. They can be jealous of the amount of love you receive in your family circle. Depending on the type of connection you have with such people, the energy of their jealousy enters your energy system through your second, third, or fourth chakra. The energy of other people's sexual jealousy affects the health of your second chakra; fellow work and academic colleagues can send you their jealousy through your third chakra; and people who are jealous of the amount of love you have in your life will send this jealousy to your heart through your hands and up your arms. The physiological effect of this energy transfer creates tension, tightness, hardness, and a slight coldness in whichever part of your body it is found.

Sibling and spousal jealousy enters your energy system at the outer edge of your hipbone, causing you to feel pain and stiffness on the outside of your hip and down the outside of your leg. In extreme cases this energy can make it difficult for you to walk. In general, the energy of the jealousy of a brother or husband will enter your energy body through your right hip, whereas the energy of the jealousy of a sister or wife will enter your energy body through your left hip.

Most people are unaware of third-party jealousy and so are unaware of the adverse effects this has on the body. If you suspect anyone in your life is jealous of you, seek the help of someone trained to see energy, such as an energy worker, a spiritual worker, or a clairvoyant, and ask if they can see any of this energy in you. An experienced energy worker

or spiritual healer will also be able to help you release this energy from
your body.

## *Loneliness*

Loneliness is more than just an emotion; it is also a longer-lasting
feeling—a mood, a state of mind, or a state of being. Regardless of what
words people use to describe what loneliness is, at the heart of loneliness
is an energy that comes from an environmental experience, such as that
of abandonment, loss of love, or absence of love.

A loveless environment is a cold environment. There is nothing
warming and nurturing about it. The resulting emotional state from
experiencing such a loveless environment—loneliness—is similarly cold.
Of all the emotional energies carried in the body, loneliness is the coldest. To understand the physiological effects of loneliness in the body,
it is best to understand the effects of cold on the body. Anyone who
begins a yoga practice in a cold room knows how difficult it is to open
the body. Muscles are cold and contracted and are difficult to stretch,
warm, and release. The body naturally contracts to protect itself against
the effects of cold. Men also see the effect of cold energy on their penis
when they come out of the cold ocean or walk outside in cold weather.
Quite simply, cold energy causes contraction.

Loneliness in infancy, whether as a result of neglect, abandonment,
or a loveless home environment, causes particular parts of the infant's
body to contract in a natural act of defense or protection against the
cold energy of its environment. If this cold environmental energy is not
released in infancy, it remains stored in the body of the fledgling human
as he grows into adulthood. As long as the original cold energy remains,
so does the original core contraction caused by that cold energy.

There are two key areas in the adult body where the energy of
infantile loneliness is stored: the pelvic girdle and the hamstrings. The
intensely cold energy of infantile loneliness is the energetic cause of, or
energetic root of, contracted muscles in the pelvic girdle and contracted
muscles in the tops of the thighs, most commonly known as closed hips
and tight hamstrings. The exact location of the cold energy that causes
the hamstrings to contract is in the space between the top of the femur

and the sitting bone. When you experience this energy, it feels like a needle made of ice stuck deep into this area of your body. When you release this energy, it feels like freezing water flushing downward through the hamstrings and the backs of the legs. As you continue to release this energy, you reduce the amount of cold energy causing the contraction of the hamstrings. This is healing the issue of tight hamstrings through the process of internal energy release.

The other area of the body that is adversely affected by the emotional energy of loneliness is the region around the heart, extending into the lungs, with the breastbone at the center. This can be felt in your own body as tight intercostal muscles, or alternatively in the body of a massage client as an area of cold energy on the palm of your hand when you hold your hand over your client's heart.

If you are sensitive to energy, you may also experience the energy of loneliness as an intensely black, solid form, similar to obsidian. Sometimes it appears as solid, deep, black ice, especially in the lungs. Loneliness is both the coldest of all the energies in the body and also the blackest. Fear is also a black energy (with the softest form of fear energy appearing as black smoke), but the black of fear feels sticky, whereas loneliness does not.

## Grief

Grief is the emotion we feel after a loss. It is usually felt in the area of the heart. It can give the feeling of living in a numbing, cool, damp, gray world. Following a loss, it can become a dominant feeling, temporarily preventing fully integrating with our environment, whether at home, at work, or socially.

Grief, however, is a soft energy. In grief it can feel like we are in the thick of gray clouds or gray cotton wool. When massaging someone carrying the emotional energy of grief, it can be felt between upper breast and clavicles. The area feels spongy, soft, and slightly cold to the touch. If you are sensitive to the colors of energy, you will sense grief as having a gray color. Although the emotional energy of grief doesn't have any adverse physiological effects on the body, its presence can cloud or fog the heart completely. The good news is that it is an emotional energy that can be easily and effectively cleared and released, particularly through a series of TCM acupuncture treatments.

### Sadness, Disappointment, and Despair

Sadness is another soft emotional energy that can be found close to the heart, usually between the breast and the clavicles. Similar to grief, it feels spongy, soft, and slightly cold to the touch. Another area where the energy of sadness accumulates is in the latissimus muscle just under the ridge of the shoulder blade. This can be very painful when you extend the muscle and squeeze it, for instance during massage. Although sadness is found in the heart area of the body, the fourth chakra, it is actually an energy belonging to the third chakra, or solar plexus. If you are sensitive to the colors of energy, you will sense sadness as being yellow. A yellow emotional energy in the heart reveals an energy that has less to do with the heart and more to do with the conscious mind. It is an emotion or feeling that has become a state of mind or a state of being.

Disappointment is very similar to sadness in terms of what its energy feels like, its associated color, its origin, and the areas of the body it effects.

Despair is a deeply held emotion that forms toward the end of life, when a person finally realizes or surrenders to life's struggles. Despair reveals the issue or struggle in life that has caused the person the deepest sadness. My father's despair was that he didn't follow his intuition at a key moment in his life, resulting in a decision he then took that trapped him for the rest of his life.

If you are an energy worker or someone sensitive to the colors of energy, the emotional energy of despair will appear dark green or blackish green. This particular energy is a mixture of green energy, representing the heart, and black energy, symbolizing pain or blockage (more on color combinations in chapter 7). Together they reveal an energy that causes a pain or a blockage to the heart. The body areas most commonly affected by the emotional energy of despair are the heart and the groin. As mentioned, it is a deeply held emotional energy that only reveals itself after years of spiritual self-development, whether through the path of yoga, massage, martial arts, or meditation.

An important thing to note about the emotional energy of despair is that it is sometimes not related to issues and struggles in your own life, but rather to issues and struggles relating to the lives of your parents. Although the energy is present in your body, it can sometimes be an emotional energy belonging to someone else, in this case one or both of your parents. (The ways in which emotional energy gets passed from parent to child are discussed in detail in chapter 6.)

### Shame and Humiliation

Of all our emotional energies, shame and humiliation harbor the greatest potential for damage, even greater than fear, in large part because, of all the things we would prefer not to reveal about ourselves, shame and humiliation cause us to feel the greatest aversion. If we feel deep shame about something we experienced in life, it can force us to block out or consciously deny large parts of our life in an attempt to bury and hide that shame. We can even rewrite our entire personal history based on our reluctance to deal with the emotion of shame.

My own mother was deeply ashamed of certain parts of her life, particularly in relation to my earliest infancy. Her shame led her to rewrite the history of certain parts of her life, so that when in adulthood I asked my mother about her life, the stories I was told were a rewriting of her personal history: I was told non-truths.

Because we bury shame so deeply, its energy is found very deeply inside the body, close to the core, or root, of our being. It is an energy wrapped very tightly around the lowest part of the spine, between L5 and S5. When it releases you can feel a sudden freedom in the movement between the vertebrae in your lower spine. The energy of shame is also one of the energies that blocks the release of another, more deeply found form of energy close to the core of our being: the kundalini. A strong yoga or meditation practice focused on the sacral vertebrae can trigger a release of the emotional energy of shame from that part of the body, which in turn can set free a release of kundalini energy. It may be possible to trigger a release of kundalini energy in massage, but the therapist would need to be someone who has already worked on releasing their own shame and their own kundalini energy.

The physiological effects of the energy of shame on the body are small and subtle, but the mental and spiritual effects are great, as it is one of the key energies that blocks us from being free. How can we expect to be free when, at the same time, we are holding on to something shameful from the past? If you want to be free, you have to let go of the energy of shame. Even if you have completely blocked your shame from your conscious mind, the energy of it still remains stored in the body.

If you are sensitive to the colors of energy, then you can find where you store the energy of shame in your body simply by finding its color: it is a dirty, pale, salmon pink.

The experience of being completely humiliated or the fear of being completely humiliated is sometimes too much for a person to bear. It is the one feeling that can lead someone to take their own life. My father carried a great fear of being humiliated by his mother for getting something wrong, and it was this fear of being humiliated by his mother that stopped him from following his intuition at a key moment in his life, when he married my mother, and instead to make a decision to stay in the marriage, which then went on to trap him for the rest of his life. I have felt the energy and presence of my father's humiliation within me. It is deep in my lower abdomen and pelvis. Each time I connect with this energy in myself, I see my father's face. I see his tears and I feel his pain.

From my own experience of working on myself, I have grown to accept and understand the energy of humiliation. However, I have yet to find it in the body of another. Maybe I have to further develop my sensitivity to the most deeply suppressed of all our emotional energies.

## Guilt

Guilt is a feeling built on a belief, or rather, one of two beliefs: the belief you have done something wrong, or the belief that you have caused something wrong to happen. The former is what I call male guilt, the latter, female guilt. Here is a simple example of what I mean. A husband promises his wife to look after her, but he doesn't (male guilt), while the wife believes she did something to cause her husband to not look after her (female guilt).

What gives guilt its strength is the level of belief given it. The more you believe in your guilt, the more energy you give it, and the more energy you give it, the more pervasive the energy of guilt will be in your body. The difficulty is that the belief in guilt can come from either your conscious mind or your subconscious mind.

Conscious-mind guilt relates to an event that happened in your current life that can be proven or validated. Subconscious-mind guilt relates to the feeling of guilt that has been passed on to you through your ancestors; this is accumulated ancestral guilt. Depending on your belief in karma, ancestral guilt can also include accumulated feelings of guilt from your own past lives. We are born with the notion of guilt hotwired into our system. One of the great sadnesses in life is that ancestral guilt is based on the notion that somewhere, back in a very foggy past life, you either did something wrong or you caused something wrong to happen. The sadness is that, in truth, the thing you think you did, you did not actually do. This is the root of all guilt: the mistaken belief that you did something wrong.

Guilt, at its core, is a mind trick. It is a mind trick that gets you to believe in something that did not happen. One of the traps in guilt is that in trying to understand it and set yourself free from it, you often have to follow it into the realm of past lives, whether through regression, rebirthing, meditation, or some other means. The trap is that in the realm of past lives nothing can be proven.

In past-life regressions your mind will reconstruct and reconstruct seemingly different episodes from seemingly different past lives. All you end up with is an ever-increasing and unending list of things you did or allowed to happen in your past lives. This brings you nowhere remotely close to understanding guilt, never mind setting you free of it.

What you need to do to understand guilt and to set yourself free is to face your accuser. Let's say for example that in a past-life regression you discover you were a mother and that, through some actions of yours, you caused your child to die. The accusation is that you caused your child to die. And for every accusation there has to be an accuser—in this case, your own conscious mind. By accepting the accusation to be true, the concept of guilt is created. Instead stop the story and demand proof that it is true. Demand your accuser show you proof of your guilt and you will discover the truth: that the pages in the book of evidence against you are blank. There is absolutely no proof that you caused the death of your child. Your accuser made the story up and then conspired to get you to believe in it. This is the root of guilt. A story that you believe in that never happened. A mind trick.

As guilt is a mind trick, its energy is mental energy and originates in the third chakra. Its energy is carried throughout the body on one specific meridian associated with the third chakra, the gallbladder meridian. Guilt is also passed from generation to generation; the energy of which is housed in the first chakra. The release of the energy of guilt can be aided by TCM treatment of the gallbladder meridian as well as massage treatment or yoga practices that address the outsides of the legs, the outer sides of the rib cage, the tops of the shoulders, and the temples on the sides of the head.

## Shock

A discussion of emotional energy would not be complete without delving into a particular type of energy, that of shock. The experience of shock has a profound effect on the subtle energy system of the body and, by extension, on the physical body itself. There are two types of shock: experiential shock and mental shock. To help explain the difference, I offer the example of a married couple, one of whom is involved in a traffic accident while the other is at home. Let's say the husband suffers the accident while his wife is at home.

The experience of being in a traffic accident and the subsequent experience of being in the emergency room produces enormous shock in the body, the more so if the hospital experience involves surgery of some kind. Experiential shock triggers the release of the energy of shock into the body. Shock energy is very cold, black in color, and creates strong contraction in the body tissues wherever it is released. Even if the husband makes a full and speedy recovery from his accident, his

body will still hold the energies of shock relating to the original accident and subsequent hospital experiences. These energies are usually
found in the first and second chakras, resulting in physical contraction
in the muscles, connective tissues, and internal organs in most of the
body areas associated with these chakras: the kidneys, adrenal glands,
lower abdominal region, lower back, pelvic girdle, hips, thighs, and
knees, including the knee joints. Because the energy of shock remains
present in the body long after the trigger event, it means that on a very
deep level there are parts of the husband's body that are still reacting to
the accident and subsequent emergency-room experience, even though
the events have long since passed.

Physical treatment of such a person involves the massage skills of
loosening and warming tight and contracted muscles, while on the
energetic level it involves making a connection to the energy of shock
present in the body and communicting to that energy that the events of
both the accident and subsequent emergency-room experience are over,
and that nothing else bad is going to happen—it's all over. There is no
more need for the person to defend himself against these events. They
have finished. He is now safe, and he can let go. This type of connection and silent communication originates in the mind of the therapist.
The therapist generates the feeling or energy of reassurance and safety,
a second-chakra energy, in his or her touch, and through that touch
transmits the warming energy of reassurance into the body of the client. It is this warming energy that counters and melts the cold energy
of shock in the body of the client.

Following the husband's accident, word is sent to his wife inform-
ing her of the accident. Upon hearing the news, the wife also receives
a shock, a mental shock. The energy of this type of shock is also black
and cold and causes contraction in her body. The energy of shock is
carried in the words delivered to the wife. When she learns of her husband's accident, the energy of shock enters her energy system through
her ears and descends down the back of her body along her spine. If she
thinks, even for an instant, that she will lose her husband, the energy
of this mental shock triggers the release of shock from within all her
chakras, from her sixth to her first. If she is in love with her husband,

the thought of losing him will trigger the release of the black energy of shock into her spine at the back of her heart chakra, where it will cause contraction and tightness in the muscles between the shoulder blades. If she has a family with her husband, the momentary thought of losing him as the father to her children will release the energy of shock in her first chakra, causing coldness and contraction to that area of her body. If the couple has enjoyed sexual relations, the black energy of shock will also accumulate at the back of her second chakra; and if there is shared property, business, or money, it will accumulate at the rear of her third chakra. Physical treatment of the wife involves the massage skills of loosening and warming the cold, contracted, tight body areas; on the energetic level it involves a similar type of energetic connection and communication as the one used with the husband, in which she is reassured that everything is now fine.

A specific type of energy connection is needed to heal shock through massage: the energy of shock is a second-chakra energy, and when released into or found in the body it causes the second chakra— the kidneys and the adrenal glands specifically—the most damage. Therefore, the type of energy connection between therapist and the client in massage also has to be of the second chakra. This means a close, intimate contact with the person—no borders, no boundaries, no use of self-protection. A strong and full connection, with the therapist offering complete support and reassurance in their touch, is necessary. It is the warming, second-chakra energies of reassurance and support offered in massage that will release the energy of shock held in the body of the person. In this case, the more formal energies of the third chakra, which are often used in massage treatment, as exemplified by statements like "I am the doctor and you are the patient," or "If you have the condition of shock, then according to the book I have to press points 1, 2, and 3 to release it," are inappropriate approaches to releasing shock energy from a person's body. The person needs the energies of support and reassurance, in much the same way a child needs intimate parental contact, support, and reassurance following a shock, and not the energy of being held at a distance or the energy of being told they will be okay if they breathe and count to ten.

In dealing with the energy of shock in massage, it is less about what kind of treatment you offer a client suffering shock and more about the energy you use in delivering your treatment. The use of loving energy in a shock-recovery massage is also helpful, but love is an energy of the fourth chakra, whereas the energy that needs healing is of the second chakra.

## The Healing Energy of Love

Love is the energy that heals all. It is a warming, expansive energy originating in the heart area. It makes cold muscles go warm, contracted muscles open and relax, and heavy muscles lighten. It unwinds confusion and dissolves pain. It creates balance wherever it flows. It melts the ice of fear and loneliness, calms the winds of anger and hatred, and liberates the body of guilt and shame. It forgives all forms of hurt and treats everyone as equals. If able to flow throughout the body, the energy of love brings healing wherever it goes.

Love is, of course, a very powerful energy, which is why sometimes it can cause pain and discomfort. When you bring the strong, warming energy of love to a part of the body that has been frozen with cold for a long time, the effect of love melting the ice causes the body cells that are full of cold energy to change, and this process of cellular change, when strong, can cause a temporary feeling of discomfort. That's why when working with the energy of love, you sometimes need to be patient, as its heating energy can cause temporary unease.

If you do the hands-off partner exercise outlined in chapter 1, you can experience the energy of love as heat on the palm of your hand when you hold your hand over the heart area of your partner. You may also experience a tingling from the center of your armpit. This latter experience is an energizing of the heart meridian. If you place your hand on the heart area of your partner, it will also feel warm or hot. This is the heat of the fire energy of love. In a massage treatment, if you feel this energy in the heart area of your client, use all your skill and knowledge to stimulate the presence of this energy, then spread it around as much of your client's body as possible in the way you spread soft butter on bread. There is nothing more healing for the body, mind, and spirit than healing with the energy of love, both for you and for your client.

If you are sensitive to the colors of energy, you will find that the energy of love is green. Not yellow green, bright green, or dark green, but rainbow green. A great form of self-healing is to imagine this color in your mind and then using your awareness, bring this color to parts of your body that you know to be in discomfort. Some people are able to imagine the color gold along with green when they do this exercise. This is a slightly more powerful color combination to use in self-healing through the use of color (a subject explored in detail in chapter 7).

The energy of love and, by extension, the energy of the heart are closely connected to the energy in your hands. There is a small energy center, or chakra, in the palm of your hand through which the energy of love can be transmitted and received. If you have a strong and open heart, there is a good chance you also have soft and warm hands. You can use warm hands to bring great healing, either to yourself or to another, by simply placing your hands on a body area that is in discomfort and simply allow the heat of the energy in your hands to melt the discomfort away. Although the act of healing hands on a partner is a beautiful thing to give, just be aware that sometimes you may cause your partner a little discomfort, or cause a tear to well up in your partner's eyes, as the heat of love melts the cold hardness of pain.

Sometimes a person with a strong and open heart can have cold hands. This is because someone in that person's life is in pain and is sending the pain to that person for healing. The other person transmits the cold, hard energy of pain into the person through the energy centers in the palms of their hands, causing their hands to become temporarily cold. When this energy is sent with great force, it can enter the person's hands through the chakras in the palms and travel up the arms and toward the heart, causing areas of blockage, resistance, and pain throughout the person's arms, including the elbows.

You may ask *What is love?* Love is many things, both simple and complex, both visible and invisible. Simple love is when a feeling of love for someone spontaneously wells up inside you and you need to share that feeling with the person. In some instances you share this love by saying "I love you" or by giving the person a big, loving hug. These actions are done spontaneously and given freely, without any need of reciprocation. You just share and give love freely. You don't need to be hugged or told "I love you" back. The energy of love causes you to give and share without condition. This is love in its simplest, unconditional form.

Unconditional love is simply that: love without conditions. Some people have an idealized concept of unconditional love as love given without conditions, yet they harbor enormous conditions, mainly that it be everlasting. Yet for love to be unconditional, it has to be free of *all* conditions, including the condition of duration. Unconditional love, therefore, must be free to last however long it lasts, whether that be a moment, a minute, a month, or a lifetime.

Complex love is quite different from simple love. Some people share love with the condition that you share it back. When they say "I love you," they want to hear you say "I love you too" in return. This is giving and receiving love, love given on the condition of receiving. This works perfectly well as long as both people's understanding of love and expectations of love are the same, when what I feel when I say "I love you" is the same as what I expect you to feel when you hear me say "I love you"; when what I feel when you tell me "I love you" is the same as what you expect me to feel when you say it. Giving and receiving are equal. Difficulty arises when two people's understanding and expectation of love are not the same, are unequal. Both your understanding of love and your expectation of love are rooted in your experience of love in childhood.

In her later years, when my mother told me "I love you," she did so with the need for me to say "I love you too" in return. The difficulty was that the love she offered was different from the love she wanted in return, and, of course, I didn't know that. The emotional feeling of love she sought from me had to match the emotional feeling of love she felt when her own mother told her that she loved her. That was my mother's subconsciously programmed understanding of what love feels like:

the way her own mother's love for her made her feel. What my mother offered me, however, when she said "I love you" was a complicated and hidden mixture of energies, emotions, and feelings. It was only years later, after my mother had died, when she visited me in a dream and told me what was in her heart when she offered me her love, that what she was offering became clear:

> Her love
> Her sadness
> Her regret
> Her anger
> Her guilt
> Her belief in not ever having enough in life
> Her loneliness

When she was alive, what my mother wanted back from me when she told me "I love you" was the same feeling of love she had once received from her own mother. Sadly, when my mother told me "I love you," I somehow didn't trust it. It just didn't feel like what love should feel like. I had a deep fear that when she said "I love you" she was asking for the right to dump all her life's pain on me, and that when I said "I love you" in return she was taking it as permission to dump all that stuff on me. When it came to love, we were completely mismatched. Mismatched love not only happens between parents and children, it often happens between adults in relationships.

After she passed, what my mother wanted from me was love in one of its simplest and most beautiful forms: forgiveness. I was prepared to offer her that, and so that was when our love began to became more evenly matched. This is the way it is with love. What it is for one person is not necessarily the same as what it is for another person. We all have different understandings of what love is, many of which are hidden from our conscious understanding of what love is. We all have different expectations of love, many of which are hidden from our conscious mind. This is why, when discussing love, it can be difficult to explain what love is, because love, for each person, is unique.

Apart from differences in the quality of love people can have in their hearts, there can also be a difference in the quantity of love people have in their hearts. The quantity of love you have in your heart and, by extension, the quantity of love you can share with another are also heavily influenced by your family upbringing. Children brought up in strongly loving environments will grow accustomed to sharing large amounts of love. For them, full-on love is the only way. They know of no other amount of love to share. In adulthood they need to be loved fully, and in return they fully love.

Children brought up in poorly loving environments will grow accustomed to sharing small amounts of love. For them, low-level love is the norm. They know of no other amount of love to share. In adulthood they are capable of giving only small amounts of love, and in return they are happy to receive only small amounts of love; they get burned out by the love of people from strongly loving environments, the strength of which overwhelms their heart and causes it to shut down. A person from a strongly loving family in partnership with someone from a poorly loving family may never feel fully loved by their partner. That's just the way it is; no one is to blame.

It can also happen that adults from very low-level love upbringings may only have enough love in their hearts to love animals. They simply do not have it in their heart to love another human being. This is never to be derided but to be honored for what it is. Similarly, some people do not have a sufficient level of love in their heart to provide the amount of love a child needs. If you only have half a gallon of gas in your tank, you cannot drive your car a hundred miles.

Love not only originates in the heart, or heart chakra, but is found throughout all the chakras, expressing itself in many different ways.

*First chakra,* familial love—love for your children, parents, and siblings

*Second chakra,* the love of pleasure—the love of going out and having fun; the love of art, artistic creation, and performance; the love of sex

*Third chakra,* the love of friendship and camaraderie—the love of communication, discussion, philosophy, and learning; the love of mathematics, logic, and form

*Fourth chakra,* the love of nature—the love of humankind; the love for your partner; the love of freedom

*Fifth and sixth chakras,* the love you have for spirits, for the dead, and for God

The list is endless. Unlimited!

### Feeling the Need for Protection?
### All You Need Is Love . . .

Protection is, in essence, a form of self-limitation. The initial feeling of a need for protection in massage work can be a valuable teacher, as it forces you to ask two important questions: first, what do I need protection from? (for example, taking on someone's bad energy or getting burned out); and second, why is this happening to me? This shows that you are not yet fully open to what you are doing and that you have some underlying block, or even fear. If this happens, don't worry. It's not at all uncommon when you first start out in massage work or as a novice yoga teacher.

When you discover and recognize the origin of your block or fear, which is always within yourself, then the block is automatically lifted. You no longer need it as a teacher, and therefore the need for protection is no longer needed. This is how you self-evolve during your massage career or your life as a yoga teacher. When you are fully open to what you are doing, your heart is open too. When your heart is fully open in massage and healing or in yoga, its energy—that of unconditional love—will allow you to transmute or neutralize any negative energy that might exist in the body of a client or student. Working with an open heart, there is no need for protection.

# The Cycle of Emotional Release
# in Yoga and Massage

Whether during a yoga practice or a massage treatment, there is a fixed, ten-stage pattern to the cycle of an emotional release of any of the aforementioned emotions. This occurs in two phases: the first phase involves a rising of the emotion, and the second phase is the resolution of the emotion. This pattern is not quite as easy to observe in yoga, as the cycle unfolds slowly, and a single class or self-practice is usually not enough time to allow the cycle to complete. But over a series of yoga asana sessions there are aspects of this cycle that can be observed.

One of the early stages in emotional release during yoga is the experience of physical discomfort that often precedes a rising emotional memory. When this happens, the temptation is often to step off the practice a little to allow any rising sense of discomfort to dissipate, while you return to your comfort zone. The other thing that sometimes happens during a yoga practice is that the overall cycle of emotional release is unintentionally broken into disjointed pieces over a series of individual practices, simply due to the nature and duration of each practice. This leaves the yoga practitioner not always able to "connect the dots" in the overall picture of what is happening, and the practitioner can sometimes be left with feelings of unease in their body that they do not fully understand.

The same cycle of emotional release can be experienced in massage. In massage, however, more time can be given to an emotional release, especially through the guiding hands of a skilled therapist, allowing an entire emotional release to pass through all its stages in a single massage treatment. In such a situation it is easy for a massage client to see how one stage of an emotional release leads to another stage of release, and to experience the different physiological symptoms that characterize each stage of the release. At the end of the massage, the person is left with a full understanding of what happened and why it happened and is not confused by any half-recognized feelings or experiences.

Through emotional release it is possible to see that seemingly different, disconnected physiological and metaphysical experiences in the body—for example, pain in the stomach, tightness in the trapezius muscle, jealousy of another person, and a mostly forgotten childhood—are actually all connected, as they are all symptoms related to a single issue or event. In this example, all the different physiological and metaphysical symptoms stem from something hidden in a long-forgotten childhood. The emotional component, or the emotional-release component, is only one link in the chain of symptoms relating to the forgotten childhood that has been causing various physical discomforts in the body of the person throughout their adult life.

## *The Ten Stages of Emotional Release*
This is an experiential description of the ten stages of complete emotional release. Each stage is characterized by different physiological or metaphysical symptoms, or effects, of the movement of energy. The journey starts with the grosser symptoms of emotional release in phase 1 and ends with the more subtle, or spiritual aspects of emotional release in phase 2. In this way it can be clearly seen how, by following the process of an emotional release, a spiritual awakening or enlightenment can be reached.

To move through one stage of an emotional release to the next, deeper stage of the release, all you need to do is just that: go deeper. Go deeper into whatever way you are presently experiencing the emotional release. If you are currently experiencing pain or discomfort, when you go deeper into it you will meet the next stage of the release coming out to meet you: an abstract sensation. When you go deeper into that abstract sensation, you will meet the next stage of the release coming out to meet you: raw emotion. When you go deeper into a raw emotion, you will meet the next stage coming out to meet you: a specific event or person that triggered the raw emotion. And so on.

There are many methods for going deeper. The way I was taught to go deeper is to focus lightly with your mind on the feeling of discomfort in your body, and while holding your focus there, move your breathing to that area of discomfort. Breathing into the area of discomfort has a metaphysical concertina effect on the discomfort. As you inhale, you hold or compress the discomfort, and as you exhale, you release the discomfort. I was taught to make some kind of reverberating sound on the exhalation to increase the release effect, a vowel sound like *oooh,* *aaah,* or *eeee.* Different teachers use different systems. All work.

Although what follows covers all the stages of an emotional release, when examined more closely it is actually a description of a release of energy rooted in an often hidden or repressed event, the presence of which is connected to a strong emotion.

## Phase I: Buildup and Release

Sometimes during a yoga practice or massage treatment, the energy of an emotion or a hidden event from the past is inadvertently stimulated, thus starting the process of buildup and release. In massage this can happen during the abdominal part of the massage. In yoga it can happen during a sequence of asanas that greatly stimulates the energy flowing through the second or third chakra areas of the body (including the second-chakra asanas cobra, boat, seated forward bend, supine bound angle, dog, cat, seated angle, balancing bear, and frog; and the third-chakra asanas bow, seated forward bend, upward boat, inclined plane, warrior I, warrior II, and half circle).

Emotional releases usually start unintentionally. For the purpose of describing the full cycle of an emotional release, I am using the point of view of a client who comes for massage who is experiencing some type of physical discomfort. During the massage, emotional energy is unintentionally stimulated, thus starting the cycle of release. I have broken the process down into ten stages:

1. **A feeling of discomfort**
   You arrive for the massage carrying some form of physical discomfort, such as swelling; tightness or hardness in the muscles, internal organs, or connective tissues; tightness in the shoulders; inflammation on the sides of the neck; or a feeling of pressure in a particular part of the body, such as your chest or head. Then during the massage, the cycle of emotional release begins.

2. **An abstract sensation**
   You begin to feel cold, heavy, tired, agitated, dizzy, nauseous,

gray or black, etc. You may begin to shiver or your breathing may change dramatically. Upon going deeper by allowing the massage to continue, this stage in the energy release shifts to:

3. **An abstract emotion**
   You begin to feel an emotion, such as anger, sadness, loneliness, or fear. The energy of the emotion is not yet developed enough to tell you what the emotion is connected to. But upon going deeper, the emotion begins to reveal its origin.

4. **Emotion with association**
   As the feeling of anger, for example, grows, something may suddenly come to you, say, a picture of your mother. If you then focus on your mother, she becomes the symbol through which you enter the next stage of the energy release.

5. **Emotion associated with a particular event**
   Focusing on the image of your mother, the event in your life relating to your mother that is causing the pain you currently feel is revealed: "Mother, you sent me away to boarding school! I hate you for doing that!" At this point there is sometimes a strong release of energy, usually an energy that has been building up inside the body for many years. The release can move you to tears, to anger, to shouting and wailing. You may have to get up and move around to help push the energy out of your body. An acute release of energy often causes muscles, tendons, and ligaments to cramp, most commonly in the hands and fingers. Foot cramping during massage is another example of an acute release of energy moving through the foot. In extreme cases an acute release of energy causes such severe cramping that it can lead to a temporary state of catatonia.

## Phase 2: Understanding and Resolution

As the first phase of the emotional release subsides with stage five, the discharge of emotional energy, the overall emotional release changes dramatically in form. Whereas stages one through five powered recognition and release—a release of discomfort, a release of memory, and a release of emotion—we enter the second phase, that of healing and understanding. In phase 2, the energy of the release now turns from releasing the past to healing the past. Almost as soon as you release the energy of a hurtful event from your past, your body needs to understand why that event happened. It needs to know the truth that lies behind that event. Seeking answers requires energy, and the energy that motivates you to find the answers comes from the continuing release of emotion in steps six through ten:

6. **The need for conscious understanding**
   "Mother, why did you send me away to boarding school?" The energy from this stage in the overall energy release drives you to find answers. The answers come as:

7. **Conscious understanding**
   "Okay, now I understand why you sent me away to boarding school. Now I can move on from this." Conscious understanding can come from asking the person who caused you the hurt to reveal the full story behind why they caused you the hurt. Alternatively, it may come through the use of additional professional help, such as counseling, psychotherapy, or family constellation work.

For most people, step six is as far as they need to go in the journey of emotional release. Following a successful series of therapy treatments, most people believe that they are now free of the event that caused the subsequent experiences of emotion, abstract sensation, and discomfort they felt in their body. However, the journey does not always end here. It is not uncommon in massage to be treating a client when suddenly they reexperience an old trauma or event they believed had been dealt with and released years ago. Now unexpectedly, in the course of a massage, it surfaces again. The truth of the matter is, it never left. Some energy relating to the original event is still present in the body. This reveals that there is still some part of the original event hiding even deeper within the person; there remains something waiting to be discovered, some part of the story that needs to be understood. The energy of the original event is still present, and now it causes:

8. **The need for a higher-consciousness understanding**

   "Oh no! Not again! I thought I had dealt with this years ago. Why is it still here? What do I do now?" Indeed, what *do* you do? If the normal process of conscious understanding is not enough to release your body of a hurtful event from your past, then you need the abnormal process, that of a higher-consciouness understanding. Here is a simplified example of one of the many ways you can get to a higher-consciousness understanding of an event that happened years ago in your life. This is the method my teacher in Chiang Mai taught me when I was seeking deeper answers to a specific event in my own past:

   - Activate the levels of higher-consciousness energy within yourself: the fifth and sixth chakras.
   - Through the medium of the energy of your higher consciousness, establish a link with the person behind the event in question (this is usually done in a semimeditative state).
   - Through the link, ask the person again the questions you previously asked them about the specific event, the answers of which brought you your previous conscious understanding of the event (stage seven).
   - Await their reply.

Activating higher-consciousness energy in your body is not that difficult. It usually involves some form of meditation. It can also be achieved with the assistance of an energy worker or spiritual healer who helps you focus your energy and awareness on the energy centers of the body associated with the higher consciousness, the fifth and sixth chakras. When these energy centers are activated, you can feel their presence in your throat and in your forehead, at your third eye. They feel like discs of energy on the surface of your skin, about the size of a silver dollar. Once you have awakened and activated higher-consciousness energy in yourself, you have the ability to connect with the spirit of another person, be they dead or alive, through that energy. It is the same process as distance healing.

There are any number of different ways to connect to another person using higher-consciousness energy. Different shamans, energy workers, or spiritual healers teach different methods of making higher-consciousness energy connections. They all work. There is no one single correct method. Regardless of the method you use in establishing a higher-consciousness connection with the person who caused you a hurt, the real importance lies in the answers you receive from that person through your higher-consciousness connection. The answers will be very different from the kind of answers you would receive in a face-to-face, real-life connection and conversation with that person. The additional information received through a higher-consciousness connection makes you see your life events in a very different light; it forms your higher-consciousness understanding of events.

9. **A higher-consciousness understanding**

Through a higher-consciousness connection, the events revealed at stage seven are now revealed to you again, but this time in a broader context and in a different light. This is your new, higher-consciousness understanding of events. This stage marks where your understanding of life extends beyond the limits set by the conscious mind. This is where you first begin to understand that a previous hurtful event in your life was part of a long chain of hurtful events that has been running through your family for generations and is not an isolated event that was designed to cause only you pain. An event that once filled you with rage is now regarded with a much deeper understanding: "Ah yes, now I see why you sent me away to boarding school."

The difference between this level of understanding and the understanding you would get in a face-to-face confrontation or through therapy is the quality of reality you attach to the hurtful event in your life. Traditional therapy tends to focus on feelings, emotions, and conscious-level understanding of the event in question; higher-consciousness therapy uses spiritual energy to reveal and understand the big picture, which includes previously hidden or unknown events. The energy of the original hurtful event at this point is transforming from the gross to the subtle. The result is that you somehow feel the event to be less real than you once experienced it. You *feel* it less. When it no longer feels real, the need to hold on to it fades. In the end, you let it go completely.

Paradoxically, although you are gaining additional information about the hurtful event in your life, it is also the beginning of the process of letting go. Seeing the big picture of the event is a direct consequence of opening your centers of higher-consciousness understanding.

10. **Spiritual understanding**

This is the stage when the complete truth behind all the events that happened in the lives of both you and your mother, which led up to her to sending you away to boarding school, is revealed. The final revelation about one's life through a spiritual understanding is, by its very nature, the antithesis of what you have believed life to be or to have been. One of the functions of the sixth chakra is to turn your understanding of life on its head. You will only understand this if you have awakened your sixth chakra. If you have not yet awakened the stores of higher-consciousness understanding and spiritual understanding to be found in your own body, by opening the fifth and sixth chakras, then the final, spiritual insights will seem completely fanciful to you.

The example I have used in this chapter to describe the full cycle of an emotional release is that of a client coming for massage whose mother previously sent him to boarding school. This fictional client is in reality me. I was the person holding discomforts and hidden emotions in my body, and I was the one who experienced this entire cycle of emotional release and healing.

## The Three Levels of Understanding

Here is a simplified version of what I covered in the previous discussion of the ten stages of emotional release, stated in terms of three levels of understanding. Using my previous example of trying to discover why my mother sent me away to boarding school, these three levels are: conscious understanding, higher-consciousness understanding, and spiritual understanding. The insights revealed in each higher level of understanding provide answers to questions that could not be given in the preceding lower level. The full truth is finally revealed on the level of spiritual communication.

Stage seven marked the level of conscious understanding of the event. This understanding resulted after a face-to-face conversation with my mother while she was still alive.

**Q:** *Why did you send me away to boarding school?*

**A:** I only wanted what was best for you. I am sorry it caused you so much hurt. Please forgive me.

A higher-consciousness level of understanding of this event came at stage nine, in which I was able to connect on this level with my mother with the help of my teacher in Chiang Mai, Jasmine Vishnu. At the time, my mother was still living in Ireland.

**Q:** *Why did you send me away to boarding school?*

**A:** I didn't want you around me.

**Q:** *Why?*

**A:** Because having you around would mean you getting to know me. I didn't want that.

**Q:** *Why?*

**A:** I did things I am ashamed of.

**Q:** *Like what?*

**A:** I cannot tell you yet. I am not ready.

I took this information into myself but never used it against my mother. What I did do with my mother was return home and ask her in person about our life together when I was young, as I had lost all memory of that part of my life with her. It took me two years to get her to open up about my childhood. All she was able to talk about was how unwell she was around the time of my birth and during early childhood.

By the time I had arrived at stage ten, spiritual understanding, my mother had passed away. She visited me in a series of dreams and meditations, bringing the final answer to my question:

**Q:** *Why did you send me away to boarding school?*

**A:** At one stage, while you were in my womb, I thought about ending my life.

**Q:** *Why?*

**A:** My marriage to your father was not working. It was a complete disaster, but I could not walk away. The only place I could go was back home. I could not do that. I hated my father too much. I could not turn back. I had to stay where I was, with your father in our marriage, but it was such a disaster. I felt completely trapped. I had to try to save my marriage. My plan was to have you. I thought that having a child would work. I thought it would make the marriage work and bring us together. Soon into the pregnancy, however, I knew it wasn't going to work. Then, when I knew things weren't going to work out between your father and me, I let you go. I gave up wanting to have you. I wanted you to leave. I even prayed for you to die. That was my plan. Because if you died, then I would have had an excuse to just be left alone. But you didn't die, so when you were born I didn't know what to do. I just didn't know what to do, and that is why I pushed you away and still push you away to this day. I had no one to help me. Your father didn't want to help me. I had no one. I was alone.

This is a such a simple answer, but one I could never have received from my mother while she was alive. By the time I began asking my mother about her past, she had been on various medications for over forty years to treat bipolar disorder. Her memory of her past was completely gone, or rewritten. There was also no way I could have received these answers in sessions of family therapy with my mother while she was still alive. It took a spiritual connection with my mother after she had passed on to finally reveal the truth.

The investigation at stage seven gave me the answer that my mother had sent me away for my own benefit. But it was the revelation at stage ten that brought me the answer that my mother had sent me away for her own benefit. This turned my awareness of this event completely upside down and released me from much pain.

The first time you attempt this journey to inner truth through energy work and higher-consciousness connection, you will need the services of a guide or teacher properly trained in energy work or spiritual work. However, once you have gone through the journey with a teacher and you fully understand it, you will be able to do it again unaided. The depth of understanding you receive about your life and about life in general is phenomenal. If you are a massage therapist, the level of life understanding you can gain from your own self-development and self-understanding will be transmitted to your client through the energy of your touch. This will allow you to give your client the opportunity, space, support, and trust to discover the same path for him- or herself.

## Emotional Release and the Five Koshas

The journey inward through the different manifestations of energy, as described above, is clearly mirrored in the Yoga Vedanta of the five *koshas,* or energy sheaths that surround the Self. We humans are like a lamp that has five lampshades over our central, pure light, or Self. Each of the lampshades is a different color and density. As the light shines through the lampshades, it is progressively changed in color and nature, such that on the one hand the shades provide the individualized beauty of each lamp, and on the other they also obscure the pure light. The yoga path of Self-realization is one of progressively moving inward through each of those lampshades so as to experience the purity

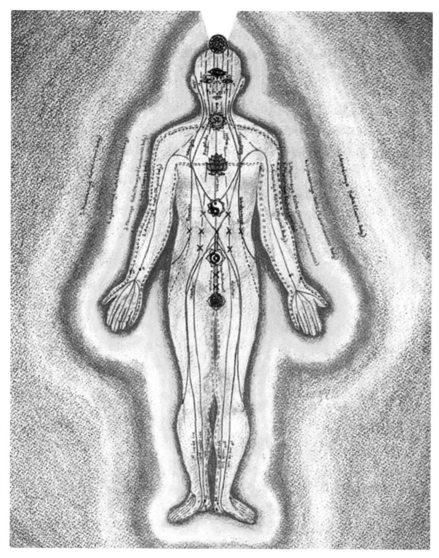

*Fig. 3.1. An artistic rendition of the chakras, meridians, and koshas*

at the eternal center of consciousness, the Self, while at the same time allowing that purity to animate through our individuality. These five levels are the koshas, which translates as "sheaths."

In figure 3.1, in relation to massage, especially Thai massage, the five koshas are illustrated by Kam Thye Chow, of Lotus Palm, in Montreal, who is one of the most established teachers of Thai massage in the West.

For the purpose of illustration, in the chart on page 124 a different color is attributed to each of the koshas.

Red is attributed to the Annamaya kosha, the physical body.

Orange is attributed to the Pranamaya kosha, the energy body.

Yellow is attributed to the Manomaya kosha, the body of memory and conscious mind.

Green is attributed to the Vijnanamaya kosha, the body of wisdom and higher intellect.

Blue is attributed to the Anandamaya kosha, the body beyond the mind, or the Spirit.

Although the koshas are shown here to be lying outside of the physical body, this too is only for the purpose of illustration. In reality, the energies to be found within each of the koshas are revealed by journeying inside, going inward, into the physical body, typically through a discipline of self-development such as yoga. As you journey inward through each manifestation of energy, as delineated in the previous section on the ten stages of emotional release, the energy you encounter corresponds to one of the koshas. To illustrate this point, I use the same five colors used by Kam Thye Chow to match my description of the ten-stage journey through the various manifestations of energy in the body, from initial manifestation to final revelation of truth and resolution.

1. A feeling of pain or discomfort in a particular part of the body.

2. An abstract sensation: you begin to feel cold or heavy, light, or tired.

3. An abstract emotion: you begin to feel angry or fearful.

4. Emotion with association: as your anger grows, you may suddenly "see" someone.

5. Emotion associated with a particular event: "You sent me to boarding school!"

6. Need for conscious understanding: "Why did you do that to me?"

7. Conscious understanding and forgiveness: "Okay, now I understand."

8. Need for higher-consciousness understanding: "Oh no, not this again! What do I do now?"

9. Higher-consciousness understanding: events revealed again in a broader context.

10. Spiritual understanding: the complete truth behind all events is revealed.

The point I wish to illustrate here is that the yogic path toward Self-realization can also be attained through the full examination of energy in forms of bodywork such as ayurveda, lomi lomi, martial arts, shiatsu, or Thai yoga massage, as well as other disciplines. All approaches lead to the same goal.

## Letting Go and Finding Balance

By journeying in through the layers of your energy, you end up letting go of much of your life's baggage and finding true balance in life. But in reality you do not let go of anything; rather, what happens is that the world lets go of you—in other words, the world has less of an effect on you.

In the beginning, when the need to journey starts because of the physical, mental, or emotional pain of your circumstances, it is as if your entire universe is defined by the sum of these day-to-day painful experiences. By journeying inward, your universe widens and expands. And as it does so, and as you take in new sensations, new teachings, and new understandings, you achieve a greater balance in life, and the impact of what was once painful in your life reduces in strength.

Using our previous color scheme as an illustration of the journey, we start out without an understanding of life's events, a state dominated by the pain of unawareness (red). As we journey progressively inward, toward the true, authentic self, the pain of incarnate life gradually is replaced by deeper levels of awareness, such that we arrive at a state of balance (the five colors, or koshas, in balance), as illustrated on page 124.

**Physical**

Pain = 100 percent of your universe and focus.

**Physical** | **Energy**

Pain = 50 percent of universe and focus.

**Physical** | **Energy** | **Memory and Conscious Mind**

Pain = 33 percent of universe and focus.

**Physical** | **Energy** | **Memory and Conscious Mind** | **Wisdom and Intellect**

Pain = 25 percent of universe and focus.

**Physical** | **Energy** | **Memory and Conscious Mind** | **Wisdom and Intellect** | **Spirit**

Pain = 20 percent of universe and focus.

*As we move toward balance in the five koshas, we lessen our identification with the physical body, a state dominated by the pain of unawareness.*

# 4

# Sexual and Karmic Energies

## Sexual Energy

Sexual energy is a second-chakra energy, the chakra that governs movement. It has many different uses, most obviously in the way we use it in all aspects of expressing sexuality, such as in initial arousal and flirtation; in sexual self-confidence; in what we find sexually attractive in a partner and how we attract a partner to us; in the chase, fun, games, playfulness, and excitement leading up to a new sexual relationship; and, of course, in the multilayered pleasures of the sexual act itself. Sexual energy also governs all aspects of fertility, conception, pregnancy, and childbirth.

Second-chakra sexual energy, however, is much more than the expression of sexuality:

- It is the energy that you use in massage or yoga when it is your intention, as a therapist or teacher, to move the energy in the body of your client or student.
- It is healing energy, necessary in the healing of another person's sexual energy.
- It is ancestral energy, i.e., that which binds us to our parents and grandparents and beyond.

- It is karmic energy, i.e., that which connects us to certain people in our life as a result of our past lives.

## The Natural Characteristics and Uses of Sexual Energy

As sexual energy belongs to the second chakra, the best way to understand the natural characteristics and uses of sexual energy is to understand the natural characteristics and uses of the energy of the second chakra, which relates to a specific stage of development in life. This stage of development is early childhood, from the time a child first walks to the age of around twelve years (although this time frame is a generalization and not an absolute). During this time of life a child's main developmental needs are related to movement, curiosity, sense-based experience of the world, creativity, fun and playfulness, innocence, and being open to giving and receiving without judgment or expectation. There are two other related emotional energies housed in the second chakra: excitement and anticipation. These are all qualities that relate to the expression of sexual energy. The overall quality of energy received in childhood for these developmental needs determines the health and balance of a person's second-chakra energy later in adulthood. When we want to keep our sexual energy in a healthy state, we should express and share it in ways that reflect these second-chakra qualities.

### Second-Chakra Energy as a Base Energy in Bodywork and Yoga

The use of second-chakra energy in yoga or massage is essential. Second-chakra energy is the energy that governs all forms of movement. It is the physical energy you use to do things. If you move your body or cause another person to move their body, you are using second-chakra energy, part of which is sexual energy. Second-chakra energy is the base energy in teaching any form of bodywork or body movement. This base energy, however, needs to be mixed with another type of energy to give the bodywork or yoga an overall style and quality.

- Second-chakra energy mixed with third-chakra, rational, intellectual, academic energy gives rise to a style that is structured, i.e., easy to follow, learn, reproduce, and is always done by the book. It represents a goal clearly defined and the path to that goal clearly set out.
- Second-chakra energy mixed with fourth-chakra energy gives rise to a style that is empowering, freeing, empathetic, sharing, loving, and understanding. In teaching, often no textbook is used or lesson plan followed. It is the energy that holds a classroom of people together so that a feeling of family is engendered.
- Second-chakra energy mixed with sixth-chakra, spiritual energy gives rise to a quality of bodywork and teaching that unveils the deepest of truths, challenges commonly accepted knowledge, triggers inspirational thoughts and dreams, and goes to the core of your being and reveals the hidden destiny inside you. Often the effects of sixth-chakra bodywork and teaching take months to filter down into the awareness of the client or student.
- Second-chakra teaching energy mixed with second-chakra energy gives rise to a style that is creative, playful, sensual, pleasurable, fun-loving, exciting, and full of laughter. It is no wonder that second-chakra bodyworkers and yoga teachers are usually the most popular and most sought-after!

Note that the exchange of massage energy or teaching energy for sexual energy is a very common occurrence in massage and other practices including yoga. This reveals a misunderstanding and misuse of sexual energy and leads to further confusion and blockages in the energy of the second chakra, the seat of sexual energy. Watch out for the massage therapist or yoga teacher who doesn't want to charge you for their services. I know of a woman who agreed to a series of treatments from a "spiritual" massage therapist who insisted on taking no payment because, he argued, it was his calling to give healing without payment. After two months of treatments, he suddenly demanded sex. She was incensed and so was he when she refused him. This is why money can be so important in massage practice and yoga. An agreement to pay money in return for massage or teaching is clear-cut and easily understood by both parties. There are no hidden extras. Always insist on a prepaid monetary agreement with a massage therapist or a yoga teacher you do not know. It keeps things clear.

## Ancestral Patterns in Sexual Energy

The sexual energy your father used to conceive you contained a microcosm of the energies of his own life up to the time of your conception, including his own experiences of life, his beliefs in life, his behaviors in life, and his emotional experience of life. If your father had a lonely childhood and it was an experience he never told you about or was never able to let go of, a microcosm of the energies of that entire experience in his life got passed on to you—in other words, your father passes a second-generation copy of the energies of his secret lonely childhood into you at the time of your conception. This means you grew through childhood into adulthood carrying a subtle version of the energies of your own father's childhood in your body. Not only is a copy of your father's genetic make-up passed on to you at conception, so too is a copy of his subtle-energy body, formed from the totality of all his energetic, emotional, and mental experiences in life.

The same applies to your mother. She too passed on a copy of the totality of her life-experience energy to you at the time of your conception. This is why, as an adult, you can sometimes feel angry or lonely, yet when you examine your life you find you have no reason to be angry or no reason to feel lonely. Everything in your life is actually going quite well. The anger or loneliness you feel is not yours, it is a subtle, second-generation copy of the anger or loneliness of one or both of your parents.

Before you take this information and use it to blame your parents for all your anger and loneliness, pause to consider that you too will pass on a copy of the totality of your life-experience energy to your own children at the time of their conception. And the totality of your life-experience energy includes a second-generation copy of the totality of your parent's life-experience energy. This is the way ancestral energy works. This is the cycle of life. Everybody is in it. The energy of the totality of life experience is passed from one generation to the next generation—parents, grandparents, et al.—through sexual energy, the energy of the second chakra, energy that is carried throughout the body in the kidney meridian and the meridian paired with the kidney meridian, the urinary bladder meridian.

The other important consideration in understanding any energetic connection between you and your parents is that any such connection is two-way. An energetic connection between you and a parent is actually a pair of connections, one that joins you to the parent and one that joins the parent to you. On the death of a parent this connection breaks, although the accumulated energy resulting from the connection up to the point of death remains in your body. You may think it is easy to break any connection that exists between you and your parents by walking away from your parents. Yes, you can break your physical connection to your parents in this way, but if the energetic connection still exists, you will remain tied to them.

## How Your Feelings about Having Children Are Predetermined

Most adults who want to be parents conceive children because they want to have children. When you were conceived, you were probably conceived with the energy of "I want to have children," or "I am happy to have children." A copy of this energy was then hotwired into your own sexual energy, giving form to your own innate feelings about having children later in adulthood. However, not all parents are happy about having a child when they conceive. Some parents feel they are being bullied by their partner or trapped by their partner into having a child. This leads to conflicted feelings and energies at the time of conception.

My own father had the intuitive feeling that it was wrong to conceive me, but he nevertheless did so as he thought the alternative would have led to marital collapse, which would have brought too much humiliation on him. My father didn't really want to conceive me, so I was conceived with the energy of "I don't really want to have a child." I then carried a second-generation copy of this energy in my own life, and this has been a hidden influence in my own decision to not have any children. The feelings your parents had about having you at the time of your conception go on to form your own feelings about having children.

### Inherited Patterns of Attraction

If you are male and your mother seduced your father, the energy with which she seduced him becomes the energy you are most attracted to and most vulnerable to in women in your adult sexual relationships. If this is the case, you will be happier in being seduced in your sexual relationships. If, on the other hand, your father seduced your mother, you will naturally be the seducer in your own sexual relationships, and this seductive energy will be what your sexual partners find most attractive in you.

The same is true if you are a woman. If your mother seduced your father, you will naturally be the seducer in your own sexual relationships, and the type of energy with which your mother seduced your father will be the energy men find most attractive in you. If your mother was seduced by your father, you will be happier in being seduced in your sexual relationships, and the energy your father used in seducing your mother will be the energy you are most attracted to and most vulnerable to.

### The Sexual-Energy Relationship between Mother and Child

Some mothers lose a lot of sexual energy during the process of conceiving, carrying, and giving birth to a child. Giving birth can leave some women feeling exhausted and completely depleted. Some mothers, before delivering their child, may have received strong feelings of self-confidence from their sexual energy. They may have loved feeling sexy. Some may have consciously used their sexual energy as a source of power to gain advantage. When such a mother gives birth to a child and realizes she has lost all her confidence-giving sexual energy in childbirth, she forms a subconscious need to have that sexual energy returned; she naturally wants back what has been taken away from her.

And subconsciously she wants it back from the person she believes took it away from her: her child.

This is why, in some mother-child relationships, the underyling subconscious need in the relationship is not a love-based one, but is rather a sexual, energy-based one. The mother's need to have her sexual energy returned to her becomes an unfulfilled frozen need that underpins the entire relationship between her and her child throughout their lifetime. This is why in some mother-child relationships it is impossible to find an emotional love-energy connection between a mother and a child. The mother thinks she needs the love of her child, but unknowingly, subconsciously, she wants the child's sexual energy instead. The child, not knowing this, gives his love to his mother believing it is his love that his mother is looking for. He has no idea she is looking for sexual energy. This can be very emotionally confusing and can result in a painful mother-child relationship.

The good news is that healing this type of mother-child relationship is surprisingly easy (for an additional discusson of this subject, see "Breaking Energetic Connections with Your Parents" on pages 188–90). If you believe you are the child in such a relationship, seek out a properly trained shaman, energy worker, or spiritual healer who can help you establish a higher-consciousness energy connection to your mother, and through this connection send her sexual energy that is pure and healthy in form. This can be done by using the metaphor of color to describe sexual energy, and sending your mother orange energy. And if you are a mother and you feel you are in such a relationship with your child, seek out a similar guide or healer, and through a higher-consciousness energy connection ask your child to send you some orange energy. And don't worry, this won't hurt or tire your child.

## Sexual Energy and Karmic Energy

It is not unusual to find it hard to let go of a former sexual partner with whom you have had an intense sexual relationship. It may be that the relationship ended many years ago, and you don't see that person anymore, yet he or she sticks in your mind.

When you have a previous sexual partner you cannot let go of completely it can reveal that there is something yet to learn about that person—what the person symbolizes in your life and what life lessons that person has brought to you. Learning such lessons is not a conscious process, however. You cannot go back to your old lover and ask, "What is the hidden life lesson between us?" Your ex-lover won't know. The answer is, after all, hidden. The way to understand a karmic connection between you and a former sexual partner is through some form of higher-consciousness connection, meditative connection, or spiritual connection. You need a guide or teacher experienced in energy work or spiritual work to help you through such a process.

The answers to karmic sexual connections are nearly always irrational or unbelievable. For example, if you have been badly hurt by a former sexual partner, maybe through sexual betrayal, it may transpire that the karmic reason for your relationship was so that your partner could take revenge on you for a hurt you caused them in a past-life relationship. When you find the hidden karmic connection in such a relationship, then the lesson you need to learn from that relationship has been learned, and so you can let go of the connection and be set free of that particular former partner.

## Karmic Energy

Karma is the energy of unfinished business from the past. This energy is stored in the body, lying dormant until its need for release. The energy, when released, reveals a story or vision in your imagination. Its purpose is to tell you an unfinished story from one of your past lives that needs resolution, setting you free to continue your spiritual journey toward full self-realization.

What I have learned from the experiences of karma stories in my massage clients is that bad things happen to good and innocent people. There tends to be a belief, when it comes to karma, that if something bad is happening to you in this lifetime, it must be because you did something bad in a past lifetime and now that karma is catching up with you. When it comes to karma, bad things can happen to good people too.

The point of karma is not to judge whether you have been or continue to be good or bad, it is merely to reveal a story, an event from life. Once the story has been revealed and the life lesson learned, then that part of your karma has been cleared and you are free to move on.

I was once treating a client for a pain she had in her right forearm. In the middle of the treatment, in my mind's eye I suddenly saw the clear picture of a homestead in early twentieth-century America. An arid region, maybe Nevada or Colorado. There was a well on the homestead, similar to the traditional stone-walled well you see in old cowboy movies. Suddenly my client appeared in the vision as a young girl living on the homestead. She was coming out to fetch a pail of water from the well and as she did so she grazed her right forearm on the rim of the wall of the well. It then transpired that the graze became badly infected and would not heal. The infection got worse and worse until eventually a doctor had to come to the homestead to amputate the forearm.

As I continued to work on my friend's arm, the face of a man appeared. I asked the man who he was and why he was in the story of the well. He confessed that he had placed a cocktail of poison made from snake venom and local poisonous plants on the lip of the wall and that when the girl grazed her arm on it, she grazed it on the poison and that is why it never healed. I asked him why he did such a thing. He initially replied that the well was the only source of water for miles around and that he was jealous that the well was on the land of the girl's family. Although this was his story, it felt to me that it was not the complete answer, so I continued massaging my client's arm. Then, after a few minutes, the man revealed that he had wanted to marry the young girl, but the girl's father refused him permission, so he poisoned the well as an expression of his dissatisfaction and in an act of revenge. With that the vision ended. The story was told and my friend was free to move forward.

Karmic revenge played an important part in the life of my own mother. The object of her revenge in this lifetime was her father. In a previous lifetime he was her twin brother, who abandoned her while they were together in the womb, leaving my mother to be born alone and to go through life on her own. That left her angry.

In this lifetime, however, her father was wise to her need for revenge on him and he thwarted her efforts completely. On a hidden, subconscious level this made my mother doubly angry, an anger she never consciously understood and an anger she deeply internalized and which negatively impacted her mental wellness.

By the time she was twenty-four, my mother found herself trapped in a loveless marriage, with a child, me, and her need for karmic revenge unresolved. It was not the life she had wanted. My mother's greatest despair in life was not understanding why her life did not work out. Sadly, she had to die and pass over to spirit before she realized the answers. Sometimes the reasons for your life not working out are hidden, subconscious, karmic ones. This is why it is always useful, if you are seeking answers to life's difficulties, to seek out the services of an appropriately trained shaman or spiritual healer. Ask them to help you discover who your karmic family is and to see if there is any unfinished business therein that needs resolution in your current lifetime.

## Using Sexual Energy in Massage to Find a Karmic or Past-Life Partner

If you are a massage therapist who is drawn to helping and healing others, mostly people of the opposite sex, it may be that you are looking for someone in particular, someone whom you have not met, yet someone who, when you do meet them, will make everything fall into place—a karmic or past-life partner. This is how this dynamic works: You may find that in your massage work you take on the shit of your clients, but at the same time you are not happy about taking on the shit of your clients. In this instance, taking on the shit of a client shows you are looking for someone. In looking for someone, you are unconsciously opening yourself to receiving. Your client unconsciously feels this in the energy of your touch, and subconsciously believing that they are the person you are looking for, offers you their shit for you to receive. You initially take on this shit, but then you realize you are not happy taking on this shit because it is not the right shit, i.e., it is not shit from the right person.

When you do find the right person in the course of your massage work, you suddenly change to being 100 percent open and happy to take on that person's shit. You intuitively know what their shit is. You know you will be able to take anything and everything this person can throw at you because you also know that you can easily cope with all their shit. Their shit fits. It's the client you have been searching for, and on a deep, spiritual level you know who this person is. Often there is a feeling that you have been connected to this person through many past lives. During the massage you intuitively know what type of healing this person needs, and you instinctively know exactly how to give it to them. You are able to heal the person fully, easily, and quickly.

Although this can happen with a real-life client in a real-life massage situation, what has really happened is that the client has become the symbol of your hidden internal female, or male, side, and they represent the way for you to reconnect with this hidden, believed missing or lost side of yourself. Although your client is symbolically revealed to be the person you have been looking for, it does not necessarily follow that you need to ask this person out on a date or get to know them as a friend, let alone marry them and spend the rest of your life with them. The person is still your client, who just happens to symbolize something much deeper.

This journey is illustrated in the story of Cinderella, wherein the prince visits every woman in the kingdom in the hope of finding the right one whose foot fits Cinderella's slipper. It is a journey that takes time and energy, and the prince has to try the feet of many women before he finds the right one, who, oddly enough, is a woman he does not initially recognize. Upon finding Cinderella, everything fits. His search is over. It is a beautiful story about the reconnection of the internal male and female within the self.

The Cinderella tale reveals the hidden role of many of your massage clients. Although they take on the physical form of being just another person coming to you for massage, what they spiritually represent is a means for you to reconnect with some part of your own inner self that has become lost, forgotten, or hidden. The way you work with your clients determines the way you will reconnect to the hidden aspects of yourself. This is a hidden reason for using sexual energy in massage: to reconnect to yourself.

## How Sexual Energy Gets Hurt

There are a number of ways in which second-chakra sexual energy can become hurt or damaged. In this chapter I will cover all the various ways in which this happens, and I also include a body map, at the end of this chapter, with a detailed description of the locations of the various forms of sexual-energy hurt in the body.

To begin with, a common way in which sexual energy is hurt is through overuse. Although sexual energy has many different constructive uses, mentioned earlier, it does not follow that you can use it to fulfill *all* its different uses. It is a finite form of energy, like battery energy. When you overuse it, you exhaust its supply, in the same way a battery becomes depleted when overused. Interestingly, the same thing happens to intellectual energy, associated with the third chakra. It is almost impossible to win both the Field's Medal and a Lasker Award in the same year; it makes more sense to choose one or the other for your intellectual energy use, but not to try to use your energy for both. Similarly, to use your sexual energy responsibly, it is best to channel it and limit its use. For example, it is very hard on your body to use sexual energy for both healing work and for regular sexual activity. If you try to do too much with it, you will exhaust both it and yourself.

Another way in which sexual energy gets hurt in women can occur during pregnancy, through the loss of a child while in the womb or through miscarriage or abortion.

In short, any time we express or share sexual energy in any way other than through its natural characteristics, we alter, change, control, corrupt, enslave, and otherwise hurt our sexual energy. If we use it in ways it is not meant to be used, over time this can lead to great anguish in the body.

The following are some common examples of the misuse of sexual energy:

- Using the number of times you have sex as a measure of how much your partner loves you
- Having sex to make you feel fulfilled
- Using your sexual energy to make other people happy
- Using your sexual energy to draw attention to yourself, when the attention you seek is not sexual
- Having sex with a need for connection
- Having sex with someone out of a sense of pity for that person
- Having sex in order to gain feelings of security
- Having sex in order to gain peer acceptance or group acceptance
- Having sex for money
- Sex in return for access to power or position
- Offering sex in return for spiritual awakening
- Sex in return for an offer of work or work promotion
- Sex in return for fame or notoriety
- Sex to relieve feelings of boredom
- Sex to relieve feelings of loneliness or emptiness
- Sex as a means to dissipate feelings of anger or frustration
- Sex as a means of taking revenge on someone else
- Sex as a way to cause envy or jealousy in others
- Sex as a means of entrapment
- Sex as a form of punishment
- Sex as a statement of entitlement, right, or ownership
- Sex as a means of exerting your sense of authority or superiority (as in believing it is your right to take sex from whomever you want)
- Sex as a reward for who you are, what you do, and what you have accomplished (e.g., healers, massage therapists, and yoga teachers who engage in this behavior)

In short, if you a) have sex for a reason, b) have sex with an expectation of receiving something else in return for it, or c) have sex in order to fill a subconscious need, you are putting conditions on the expression and sharing of your sexual energy. Conditions placed on the use of sexual energy mean sexual energy is not free. This causes pain and hurt in one's sexual energy, pain and hurt that gives rise to physiological experiences of pain and hurt in certain areas of your body, as will be discussed later in this chapter. If your misuse of sexual energy is chronic or long-term, you not only make yourself ill, you can make your sexual partner ill in the same areas of their body when you have sex with them.

## Sex "on Tap"

There is one way in which we put a condition on sexual energy that causes great anguish, and that is when we expect it to be there all the time, anytime we want it—to be "on tap," as it were. This is not the way sexual energy works. In the same way kids in the playground spontaneously meet and play with other kids and then leave and walk away from them when it is time to go home, so it is with sexual energy. It is free, immediate, and spontaneous, yet we must be equally free to lose interest and walk away from it whenever we wish. We tend to think something is wrong when we lose sexual energy or sexual interest. Yet there is nothing wrong with this. It's normal. It is not normal to believe that sexual energy should make us sexually available and active 24/7, for however many years. You can see the amount of anguish this belief causes our body and our energy due to the amount of stress this condition brings with it, not to mention all the time and money we spend on drugs and therapy trying to make this belief the truth. Sexual energy should be free to come and go as it wishes, in the same way a child is free to make and break friendships in the playground. Yes, we should be free to have sex, but at the same time when our sexual energy says "no," we should honor it.

## Using Sex to Feel Free

One of the great joys of sex, or in the use of sexual energy, is the feeling of freedom it brings. Remember, the energy of the second chakra, which includes sexual energy, is used to help a child through the stage of development in her life that involves movement, creativity, and a sense-based understanding of the world. The child is not yet at a stage to understand rules and intellectual reasoning. Accordingly, second-chakra sexual energy is also an energy that is without rules and reasoning. When you express sexual energy in adulthood, part of what you express is the "without rules" characteristic of that second-chakra energy, which you feel and interpret as freedom from rules, or just plain freedom. The problem occurs when some people enjoy the feeling of freedom so much that they use their sexual energy by having sex in order to feel free. This is putting a condition on the use of sexual energy. Yet sexual energy in its natural, healthy state does not contain any conditions. It is without rules. So each time you use your sexual energy, in whatever form, to feel free, you are hurting it. You are damaging the very thing that makes you feel free, and you are damaging it because it makes you feel free. Your sense of freedom should not depend on the use of sexual energy. Your sense of freedom should be just that: free. Dependent on nothing.

### Exchanging Sexual Energy for Healing and Teaching Energy

It is not uncommon in massage for a client to release sexual energy into their body with the subconscious intention of receiving extra healing energy from the therapist. When sexual energy is released by the massage client—in most cases subconsciously—the therapist responds by finding the massage more pleasurable. Upon finding the massage more pleasurable, an untrained therapist will probably become more focused in the massage or make the massage last a bit longer than their usual treatment. What is really happening is that the therapist is giving more of their healing energy to the client, whether by extending the duration of the session or by giving a more intensely energetic massage. This is what the client needed and succeeded in receiving from the therapist by releasing sexual energy into the massage. A similar situation can occur in a yoga class, wherein a student attempts, albeit subconsciously, to get more attention from the teacher.

This kind of situation reveals a person who in childhood was trained to offer their second-chakra energy, in the form of playfulness, performance, or laughter, to their parents in return for feelings of love and appreciation. This behavior then evolved into a pattern that gets triggered whenever the person senses the healing or loving energy of the massage therapist or yoga teacher and unconsciously offers second-chakra sexual energy in exchange for feelings of love, healing, or recognition.

## How to Handle the Release of Sexual Energy in a Massage Session or Yoga Class

Whether through strong asana, dynamic flow, or vigorous massage technique, sexual energy is sometimes inadvertently released during a yoga practice or a massage treatment. This may or may not be intentional. In a massage, if a client inadvertently releases sexual energy into their body, as the therapist you feel it by suddenly finding the massage a sensually pleasurable experience. You may even find yourself attracted to the person. When this happens it is not your client hitting on you; the person is just innocently, unconsciously releasing energy, which just happens to be sexual energy. When it happens, pause in the massage for a few moments, center and gather yourself, and only then continue. When you restart the massage the sensually pleasurable feeling should be broken, thus freeing you to continue your work.

Some people who have learned to offer sexual energy in return for feelings of love or healing will find it difficult to break their pattern during a treatment. This is because they are not consciously aware they are doing it. If you are working with such a person who cannot stop releasing sexual energy, continue, but with the following unspoken intention: You do not need to use your sexual energy with me to get what you need. I will give you what you need without you offering me your sexual energy to get it.

The same thing can happen in yoga. If one of your students innocently releases sexual energy into their system, you may find yourself becoming attracted to that person. This is not your student hitting on you, just a case where the person is innocently releasing some sexual energy. Take a few moments to center and ground yourself. Break the connection to the person for a moment. When you are settled, continue. Difficulty arises when a yoga teacher, lacking experience or proper awareness of sexual energy, acts on the impulse of their sexual attraction to a student. This can lead to confusion in both parties and only reinforces the damaging subconscious behavior pattern in the student.

Difficulty also arises when a therapist or teacher skilled in sexual energy manipulation purposefully creates a series of asanas, movements, or massage techniques designed to release sexual energy from the body of their client or student. Some professionals do this so they can suck in the sexual energy that has been released into their environment. They then use this sexual energy to fulfill some subconscious need. How do you know when this is happening? You may find yourself having less sexual energy after participating in a series of yoga classes with the same teacher designed to stimulate sexual energy. By contrast, some professionals do this so they can use the sexual energy that has been released into their environment to seduce someone. How do you know when this is happening? If you find yourself sexually attracted to your yoga teacher or massage therapist in their classroom or therapy room, ask yourself if you would also be sexually attracted to them if you saw them on the street, outside their professional environment. Note that you may also find yourself attracted to your teacher or therapist because subconsciously you are seeking something from them.

## Unhealthy Sexual Control in Schools of Yoga

In my massage practice I have given sexual-energy healing to students of certain schools of yoga that teach the control of sexual energy as part of its methodology. There is a difference between sexual control that is healthy and sexual control that is unhealthy. The way you tell the difference is in the color of the sexual energy present in the body of the person when they come to you for healing through massage.

When sexual-energy control is taught to a student by a yoga teacher with the hidden desire to control the body and sexual energy of the student, the color of that person's sexual energy will be dark steel gray in color. The student's sexual center will also feel cold when you hold the palm of your hand about four inches over it. This is an absolute sign of unhealthy sexual energy. Healthy sexual energy is rainbow orange in color and feels within the normal body-temperature range of cool to warm. Dark, cold, steel gray energy is the color of energy used in cults (more about yoga cult energy and cult energy in general in chapter 6).

If you are a teacher or student of a school of yoga that asks for some form of sexual control, the way to discern whether this control is healthy or unhealthy is to get the quality of your sexual energy checked by a shaman, spiritual healer, or energy worker specializing in sexual-energy healing, or get checked by a clairvoyant able to read the energies in your body. This is how you can tell the difference between yoga that is a cult and yoga that is not a cult. The energy of cult yoga is always dark steel gray, and the energy with which a cult teacher teaches is the same color. If your sexual energy is dark steel gray, you will pass this cult energy on to any other person you have sex with. This is how cults spread.

## Sexual Energy as Healing Energy

Sexual energy in its form as healing energy is a wonderful and beautiful energy to behold. You can feel its presence in some people—mostly women who have the gift of sexual healing. It feels cool in temperature, soft and fuzzy to the touch, gentle in nature, soft black in color, and yielding, supportive, and deep in its strength. It is tremendously healing in effect. When you connect with a sexual-energy healer, their energy supports you in the same way the sea supports your body weight when you float in it, supporting you for as long as you need to be supported. You feel suspended in energy, healing energy.

Sexual-energy healing can also occur in dreams and meditations, in which the healing energy takes the symbolic form of a female figure. She sometimes appears as a woman with black hair, other times wearing a black bra or other black undergarments. Black represents yin, female, sexual-healing energy. If you see the female figure with black hair, it symbolizes that the energy she is bringing you will bring a healing to the energies of your sixth chakra. If you see her wearing a black bra, it symbolizes energy that will bring a healing to the energies of your heart chakra. If you see her wearing black panties, it symbolizes energy that will bring a healing to the energies of your first chakra. If you ever see such a symbol in your dreams, it reveals the presence of a very healing energy coming to enter your energy field. If you wish to take advantage of such a healing energy, give recognition to the female figure you see in your dream. Talk to her, introduce yourself to her. If you do not give her recognition, she will assume you have not seen her and will leave. She visits both men and women in dreams.

If you ever have such a dream and you recognize the female in black coming to bring you healing, it may be that you have previously been kind to this person and now she is coming to you in your dreams to thank you and to offer healing to you. She is doing this through the use of her sixth-chakra energy. It is a totally unconscious act. She has absolutely no conscious awareness that she has visited you in a dream to bring you healing. If you ever see this person in the real world, it is advised you do not mention your dream, as telling her could be misleading to your friend.

Another symbol through which female sexual-healing energy presents itself in dreams is the symbol of the Lady of the Lake, a potent dream symbol described in chapter 2 (pages 37–38), an archetypal figure involved in healing of both the first and the second chakras.

It may seem fanciful that you can receive sexual healing while you sleep at night, alone in your bed. You can. Certain energies, higher-vibration energies, energies belonging to the sixth chakra, transcend the limitations of our consciously perceived three-dimensional world. They transcend time and space, connecting people over long distances. Such energies can travel through people, connecting minds but not bodies. Distance healing and astral travel are two additional examples of the transcendent quality of sixth-chakra energy. Sexual healing in dreams, which is a form of distance healing, is another.

Sexual-healing energy transmitted and received through dreams reveals an important truth about sexual healing: you do not need to have sex with a person, or even touch the person sexually, in order to heal them sexually. One of the worst misuses of sexual-healing energy is the way in which it is sometimes used by healers or teachers as an excuse to have sex with a client or student. As a therapist or healer, it is your role to heal your client, not to have sex with the person on the false pretense of sexual healing. That is rape. As an energy healer, it can be part of your role to cleanse a client's sexual energy of past hurts, so that their future sexual relationships will not cause further hurt. It is not your role, however, to be that future sexual relationship. That is the role of someone else.

### Healing Hurt Sexual Energy in Massage

Sexual-healing energy can be transmitted in a healing massage treatment to bring healing to those parts of a client's body that have been hurt sexually, for example in a woman's body following a miscarriage or abortion. The color of energy used when normally touching another person in massage is orange; this is second-chakra energy, and it naturally contains elements of sexual energy. The color of the energy used in sexual healing is soft black, so in a sexual healing massage, the therapist needs to use a mixture of orange and soft black energy. There is no element of sexual arousal, flirtation, game playing, or fun in soft black energy, which of the two colors should dominate during the massage.

In sexual healing massage you begin by first tuning in to the sexual energy of the person. From my own experience, this does not start out as a conscious intention. It happens spontaneously, which is in keeping with the natural way of sexual energy. During the massage you will sense some form of sexual healing may be about to happen when you first feel a slight sexual stimulation in your own body. This reveals the connection to your client's sexual energy. As soon as you notice the slight stimulation, pause the massage to correct the balance of sexual energy in your massage, from orange, to orange and soft black, with soft black dominating. Another way you might sense your client's sexual energy is by seeing the color orange in your mind's eye. Healthy sexual energy is rainbow orange in color. Sexual energy that has been hurt is orange, but with another color, such as gray, dark gray, or black intertwined with it, like two strands of intertwined liquorice. The way to heal this hurt sexual energy is to visualize grabbing hold of the two strands of orange and black (or gray, etc.) energy and unravel the black strand from the orange, until only the orange remains. Cast the unraveled black energy away, making sure you brush off any of it from your own hands. Once you have unravelled and cast away the black energy from the orange energy, what is left is healthy, cleansed orange sexual energy. Symbolically return this energy to the body of your client. As a therapist, you need to have the relevant experience and sensitivity to differentiate between the energy of sexual healing, a soft black energy, and the energy of hurt, a cool-to-cold, slighty moist, slightly heavy, solid black energy. It is not an easy distinction to make.

Please remember that you do not need to touch or have any part of your body in contact with the body of your client while healing their sexual energy, even if the energy that needs healing is in your client's ovaries, womb, vagina, scrotum, or penis. The unraveling energy technique described above is a hands-off technique.

## Hidden Forms of Hurt to Women's Sexual Energy

Thousands of years of patriarchy have resulted in many different, more subtle patterns of hurt to women's sexuality that are not easily recognized because they have become inscribed in our collective psyche as a result of having been passed down through innumerable generations. Ultimately, these patterns hurt both women *and* men, as we shall see at the end of this chapter in the map of body hurts, and in the discussion of ancestral patterns in chapter 6. The following are just a few examples of the more esoteric hurts to women's sexual energy that I have encountered in my years as a healer.

### *Female Healers Forced to Be Prostitutes*

Throughout history there have been female healers, female priests, female seekers of truth, and female teachers of truth. This is the woman who uses her energy, including her sexual energy, for the purposes of healing and truth. Similarly, throughout history there have been males who have used magic rituals and systems of hierarchical, organized religion to build empires for themselves. The greatest threat to these power-seeking males has always been the woman who uses her sexual energy for the purposes of healing and truth.

This is the female healer who is able to see through patriarchal systems of organized, magic- and ritual-based religion. Since the basis of empire-building is control, the one thing that challenges such control is the truth. Men in these circles of magic-based religion have always understood that you cannot control the woman as healer and truth-teller, for she is free and beyond control. But you can control her as prostitute. The prostitute can be owned, controlled, and used. The prostitute poses no threat, whereas the female healer or teacher of truth does. Therefore men in patriarchal power circles have historically used magic, hexes, spells, and curses against women to block the sexual energy they use for healing and truth, while offering them "rewards" if they use their sexual energy for seduction and the pleasuring of men. In this way throughout history, women of truth and healing have been turned into prostitutes all the way up to the present. Although you may regard this as outlandish or fanciful, you can actually feel this energy process in the bodies of some women.

There are some women who use their bodies and their sexual energy as a means to get what they want in life. They know they do this, but they are not happy they act this way. They wish they could stop this behavior, as they feel trapped. Using their bodies to get what they want causes conflict, hurt, and pain. Their bodies are dense and blocked. Similarly, there are women with strongly seductive sexual energy who are tired of being recognized and rewarded only for their sexual attractiveness and not for any other aspect of who they are. These are women trapped in a way of using their sexual energy that their as-yet-unawakened intuition knows to be incorrect. Deep down inside these women are female healers whose sexual-healing energy has been blocked and subjugated by the energy of patriarchal religions. When you do healing work or energy work with such women, the subjugating male energy reveals itself by the symbolic face of its creator, or by the color silver. You can metaphysically feel blockages in the energy flow in the kidney and spleen meridians. Silver is a color attributed to an energy form of high vibration. The energy of male-conceived magic-based religion is described as a high form of energy. Its presence lies outside the normal range of sensory-based experience, which is why a woman who carries it within her energy system is unable to feel that it is within her.

It is possible to reconnect a woman who is unhappy in her imposed or unwanted role of seductress or prostitute to her original role as healer and truth-teller, to free her from a role in which men only reward her for her sexual presence and restore her to her healer role, in which she is free to be whomever she wants to be, where everyone sees her for who she truly is. This form of healing can be achieved by energy workers or spiritual healers specializing in sexual-energy healing or spell-breaking.

## Blocking Women's Enjoyment of Sex

In my massage and healing work I have found certain women, usually of great beauty and open-heartedness, to have their sexual energy blocked by the energy of some quasireligious group. The effect of this group energy is to block the woman from enjoying sex or conceiving a child. The reason for this is that the quasireligious group—always men—have "marked" the woman in her early teenage years to be a suitable woman to join their community when she is older. She is literally marked out for future use with an energy in the form of a hex or spell, which is cast into her sexual chakra and organs of reproduction. The hex energy then works to block her own independent sexual development and will only be undone when she joins the community that cast the spell.

The metaphysical effects of this kind of spell-casting is to make the organs of reproduction in the woman cold. The womb is filled with quasireligious energy, allowing no room for any other form of energy to be present, such as the energy of a child. When you do healing work with such a woman, you can see that her womb is metaphysically filled with the ghostlike faces of the men who cast the spell into her. Her sexual energy, normally orange in color, will be contaminated by an energy that is silver, which is sometimes embedded with a quasireligious symbol such as a cross or a face mask. The cross or face mask is also usually silver, silver and gold, or silver encrusted with multicolored jewels. These are all symbols of a higher-vibrating energy.

Healing a woman of such a hex is easy, but the healer needs confidence to break the will of the quasireligious group that cast the hex, along with the spiritual strength to cast out the energy of the hex. Removing the hex from the organs of reproduction returns the woman to levels of normal body heat and creates the space necessary for new life to grow.

### *Women Blocked from Conceiving by Parental Energy*

It is not unusual for a parent to be afraid of their children growing up and leaving the nest. If a parent is deeply afraid of what their life will become after the children have left, they might single out one child in particular—for example, a daughter—and pray that that child stays at home a little longer. Such a parent knows that the one thing that will take their daughter away from home is when she becomes sexually active and independent and starts her own family. In desperation, a parent may pray that she doesn't meet someone or start a family soon. If the parent is really desperate or is a devoutly religious person, or if they pray with great vigor, the energy used in the prayer can form a kind of spell, which is then cast into the body of the daughter. This is almost always unintentional, even if the results are not.

Not wanting your daughter to grow up sexually and start her own family creates a spell energy similar to a more traditional symbolic form of spell energy, such as an octopus or a chicken foot. The base energy, which is the fear of what will happen after the daughter leaves home, is black in color. The sending energy, which is a family member, is red in color. The target energy is the orange sexual energy of the daughter. This is why such a spell is black, red, and orange in color. Sometimes the ghostlike face of the parent is revealed in the red energy.

Healing a woman of this type of block involves having a spiritual conversation with the parental figure to show them they have no right to own the sexual freedom of their daughter. This needs to be clearly and lovingly conveyed in an imaginary conversation. Freedom is a sacred right bestowed on all souls, and no one has the right to interfere with this right. When the parental figure realizes this is true and accepts this truth, they release their need to keep their daughter from becoming sexually independent and starting a family.

Some parents carry a subconscious yet very strong belief that they have the right to own and control the sexual energy of their children. They are often not fully aware they carry this belief, nor are they fully aware of the consequences of such a belief in ownership of their children. It is sometimes seen in the approval or disapproval of a daughter's boyfriends. Sexual ownership by a parent of their daughter can have an invisible adverse effect on the daughter's sex life. It can influence the type of partner she chooses and how openly and deeply she enjoys the act of sex. Healing a woman with this type of blockage again involves having a spiritual conversation with the parental figure, asking them if their right to the sexual ownership of their daughter is a true right or a false right. In the conversation, they will reply that it is a true right. The parent is then asked to prove the truth supporting their right. In all cases, the parent will be unable to offer such proof of the truth and so the right to sexual ownership is revealed as false and therefore non-existent. This needs to be clearly and lovingly conveyed to the parent in the spiritual conversation. When the parent realizes that their belief in the right to own their daughter's sexual energy is nothing but a falsehood, they will release their sexual control over the daughter. This is spiritually based sexual healing, i.e., the use of spiritual energy to release an energy blockage from a woman's real-life sexual energy.

## Cleaning Your Sexual Energy

If you are a yoga teacher or massage therapist who uses sexual energy as an important part of your work, it is vital that you have the health of your own sexual energy checked on a regular basis. You can do this with a spiritual healer, an energy worker specializing in sexual healing, or a shaman. Sexual energy is a complicated energy to use and work with, and as you know from this chapter, there are many unhealthy forms and uses of sexual energy that, if you are unaware, can cause you degrees of unease, ill ease, or disease. And it's important to know that healthy sexual energy does not mean you are able to have lots of sex. Healthy sexual energy means sexual energy that is free of abuse and misuse. It is equally important to be very grounded in your work. Being strongly grounded facilitates the process of letting sexual energy from another person pass through your own energy system quickly and easily, without causing you any adverse side effects.

## The Physiological Locations of Hurt Sexual Energy

To understand the areas of the body governed by the condition of one's sexual energy, it is best to first know which areas of the body are governed by the second chakra: an area of the body that radiates from a point two finger-widths below the navel. On the front of the body, this area extends from the top of the pubic bone to the navel. On the back of the body, the area extends from L4 and L3 in the lumbar area to the tops of the adrenal glands, just below the bottom ribs. This is the area of the body directly affected by the quality of energy belonging to the second chakra.

When the overall quality of energy in your second chakra is cold, you will feel this coldness in your lower abdominal cavity as well as in the internal organs and glands associated with the second chakra: the kidneys and the adrenals. The coldness also gives rise to the experience of weakness in the muscles and internal organs in this area of the body, most noticeably the muscles that govern the bladder and support the lower back around L4 and L3. This cold feeling is often carried to other parts of the body, most noticeably downward through the pelvic girdle into the tops of the hamstrings, and further downward into the backs of the knees, on either or both of the energy meridians associated with the second chakra: the kidney meridian and the urinary bladder meridian.

People who find it difficult to enjoy the active or exciting aspects of life are normally cold in these areas of their body. So too are people who have a concept of what love is or what enjoyment is, but find it difficult to really feel and experience love or enjoyment. Indeed, these are usually people who find it difficult to feel or enjoy life in general. On the other hand, when the overall quality of the energy in the second chakra is warm, then all the organs, glands, and muscles associated with the second chakra function in a healthy state. Sexual energy additionally governs the quality of health in the body areas and internal organs associated with fertility and reproduction.

## Symptoms of Hurt Sexual Energy

The occasional misuse of sexual energy does not result in any adverse physical effects on the body. The human body can process and release from itself small amounts of toxicity and toxic energy on a daily basis. Just like having a slightly stressful day in the office, or sitting for an hour in heavy traffic without sufficient wind to blow the carbon monoxide away, the body is capable of processing and releasing small amounts of sexual toxicity without leaving behind any adverse side effects.

Continual misuse of sexual energy, however, causes the levels of toxicity that result from this damage to sexual energy to rise beyond the body's natural ability to process and detoxify. To see the most common effects of the misuse of sexual energy on the body, ask any bar girl in Thailand where their body hurts, and they will always give you the same answer: stomach and lower back. They will also say that they always feel sick. These are the three most common physiological manifestations of misused sexual energy in the body: you feel sick, your middle and lower abdomen feels cold or unwell, and your lower back hurts.

If you are someone who does not misuse their sexual energy yet you feel this way after having sex with a new partner, it may be a sign that your new partner has a strong presence of unhealthy sexual energy in their body. It is the other person's sexual energy that is causing you to feel ill.

### Sexual Energy Damaged Beyond Repair

Sadly, not all damaged sexual energy can be healed. Sometimes the hurt is too deep, the damage too corrosive. This is mostly seen when there has been a history of sexual abuse, violence, abandonment, or extreme neglect by a parental figure, most notably by an opposite-sex parent. What happens is that if you are an adult who has been the victim of acute or chronic abuse by an opposite-sex parent, you will find that in your adult relationships a time will come when you hit an enormous brick wall. Examples of this wall include:

- Not wanting to be touched by your partner
- Extreme sensitivity to all environmental stimuli
- Not wanting to start a family with your partner
- Deciding to start a family in the hope it will help your relationship, but after the birth of your child realizing that it did not work; you may even want to leave the relationship

To be fully open to your partner in relationship—in this example, a heterosexual relationship—you need to be fully open to your opposite-sex parent. This means forgiving them fully for what they did to you and loving them fully for who they are. If you are not fully open to your opposite-sex parent, when you start a relationship and open up into that relationship, you will eventually come up against the same obstacles you still hold against your opposite-sex parent. In a way it is similar to what happens to a person who is recovering from alcoholism or drug addiction. It is very rare that a person who has been severely hurt by addiction can return to a normal, everyday relationship with alcohol or drugs. The wounds from the original experience cut so deeply that if the person tries to return to using alcohol or drugs, the old wounds are reopened in short order.

In instances where the damage to a person's sexual energy is severe, the only course of healing is protection, protection from opening too deeply into a relationship. In extreme cases of early abuse, this may involve abstaining altogether from committed adult relationships involving sexual connection. It is the same as recovering alcoholics having to totally abstain from alcohol.

Healing massage and bodywork can involve releasing historically damaged sexual energy from the body, but it does not normally involve turning damaged sexual energy into healthy sexual energy. To release all damaged sexual energy from a client in massage, the client needs to be ready to release all that energy from their system. If the person is still holding on to any aspect of that energy—mostly by not fully forgiving their opposite-sex parent who hurt them—then as a therapist you cannot release that energy from their body.

## Forgiveness
## Is the Best Form of Healing

In massage, you cannot release a hurt from a client that you have not released from yourself. You cannot help a client let go of something you yourself have not let go of. You will first experience resistance, then hit an unfathomable brick wall. For example, if, as a massage therapist, you are still holding on to any unfinished business with a parent, you will encounter resistance in your massage work with the gender of any client who is the same gender as the parent with whom you still have unfinished business. When you let go and release yourself from your own pain, you can set free that same pain in the body of a massage client. When you release the client's pain, there is nothing for it to cling to on yourself, because you no longer have the receptors for that pain; you have set yourself free of it.

To let go and release any pain you are holding on to in your own body, you have to fully forgive the source of that pain. This is why the best form of protection, as well as healing, is forgiveness—forgiveness of everyone in your life who has caused you hurt. When you have forgiven and let go of all the hurt in your life, you also forgive and let go of the same hurt from all the bodies of all your clients in massage. You can no longer be adversely affected by them.

# A Body Map
# of Sexual Energy

Sexual energy is a complex energy to understand and deconstruct. Certain areas of the body governed by the second chakra, including the kidneys and lower abdominal region, house not only your own sexual energy but also the sexual energy of your former lovers and even your parents, as discussed earlier in this chapter. These energies lie in layers over one another, like the layers of an onion. As you work deeper into your sexual energy, you will discover where your body holds each of the different layers of your sexual energy history.

**First layer:** The current state of your overall sexual energy; the way you are today

**Second layer:** The sexual energy of your current or last sexual relationship

**Third layer:** The sexual energy of all your other prior sexual relationships

**Fourth layer:** The sexual energy of your first sexual relationship

**Fifth layer:** The sexual energy connection between you and your parents following your birth

**Sixth layer:** The nature of the sexual energy between your parents in the act that led to your conception

**Seventh layer:** The individual sexual energies of your parents up to the point of your conception

In figure 4.1, the orange lines very loosely reflect the runnings of the kidney meridian. The kidney meridian is the meridian associated with the energy of the second chakra, carrying that energy throughout the body along its course. This energy includes sexual energy. The gray areas reveal where the different kinds of sexual hurt and pain are held in the body. The second chakra and the organs associated with the second chakra, the kidneys, are where most of our sexual energy is housed, hence the greatest shading in those areas.

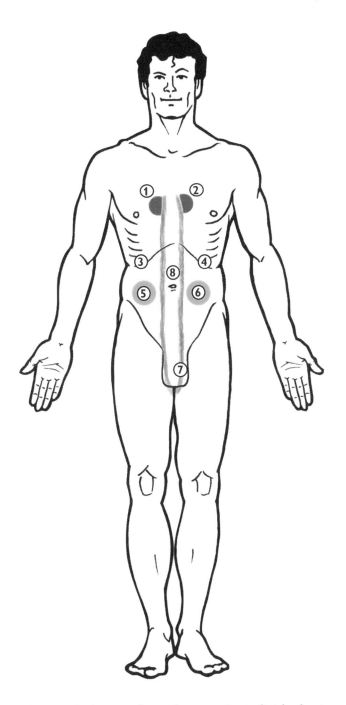

*Fig. 4.1. Body map of sexual energy. See individual point
descriptions for points 1–8.*

Traditionally, the left side of the second chakra is where we store the energy that shapes our beliefs about behavior in adult sexual relationships. The right side of the second chakra is where we store the energies of the actual experiences resulting from our adult sexual relationships. The energy housed in the right kidney is the energy we use to attract a sexual partner to us, while the energy we use in letting go of a sexual relationship is housed in the left kidney.

The following descriptions delineate the different points, 1 through 8, in figure 4.1 on page 155.

## Point 1: Kidney Meridian, to the Right of the Sternum, in the Area of the Heart Chakra

### First level of pain
The pain of using sex to avoid loneliness

## Point 2: Kidney Meridian, to the Left of the Sternum, in the Area of the Heart Chakra

### First level of pain
The pain of your heart at being controlled by your pattern of sexual behavior

### Second level of pain
The pain that comes from having one or both of your parents owning you sexually, parents who loved you only when you shared your second-chakra energy with them. You gave of your second-chakra energy in order to feel their love, for example doing a little song or dance routine for them or making a nice, big drawing for them so they will give you a hug and a little bit of love. The pain, being close to the heart, reveals the heart is not free to give and receive love. It has been subjugated in favor of the second chakra. This hidden childhood pain is revealed in adulthood by such beliefs as *You can't have love without sex* or *I need to have sex in order to feel love/loved*. This is putting your sexual needs and the unfulfilled needs of your second chakra ahead of the needs of your heart.

## Point 3: Right Kidney

*First level of pain*
The energy you use to sexually attract other people to you

*Second level of pain*
Your father's pain at being controlled by the sexual energy of your mother (if applicable)

## Point 4: Left Kidney

*First level of pain*
Pain caused by your fear of sexual energy (if applicable). Fear of sexual energy shapes your sexual behavior in adulthood. This fear can originate in the experience of being physically or emotionally abused, hurt, neglected, or abandoned by one or both of your parents, or by being sexually abused by someone in your childhood.

*Second level of pain*
Vulnerability to people who can control you with their sexual energy

*Third level of pain*
Fear of being controlled by your partner's sexual energy, for example, the fear that if you do not satisfy your partner sexually you will give them an excuse to hurt you, abandon you, or get angry with you. The fear of being controlled by your partner's sexual energy is very different from the control you impose on yourself due to your fear of being controlled by your partner's sexual energy. Although they are strongly connected, they are different types of energy. One is fear (black, yin, water), the other is self-control (yellow, yang, air). Both need to be addressed in sexual healing.

*Fourth level of pain*
Your mother's pain at being controlled by the sexual energy of your father (if applicable)

## Point 5: Right-Hand Side of the Second Chakra

*First level of pain*

The area where you store the energies of all your sexual relationships, from your current relationship, through the complete history of all your former relationships, to the first sexual relationship, which triggered the pattern of sexual behavior in all your adult sexual relationships. These energies can be loveless, abusive, hurting, or controlling and have a cooling, constricting, and hardening effect on your body. They can also be positive, nurturing, and loving and have a warming, expanding, and softening effect on your body.

*Second level of pain*

The pain or hurt from the control you impose on your sexual energy for fear of being hurt in your adult sexual relationships, as exemplified by the belief *The way I protect myself from my partner hurting me is to have sex with him/her*

*Third level of pain*

The pain of your jealousy of others in sexual union

## Point 6: Left-Hand Side of the Second Chakra

*First level of pain*

The pain of being sexually controlled by your partners in adult sexual relationships. The way you are sexually controlled by your partners may be expressed by such subconscious sexual contracts as *If you want my love, you must give me your sexual energy (have sex with me);* or *If you do not want me to hurt you or abandon you, you must give me your sexual energy;* or *If you want something from me, such as access to my money, power, or position in society, you must give me your sexual energy.* These types of hidden sexual contracts and the damaging behavior that arises from them can exist between you and your current sexual partner, former sexual partners, or the first sexual relationship that triggered the pattern of behavior in your adulthood. The pain of being sexually controlled is different from the fear of being sexually controlled, and different again from the control you impose on yourself as a result of the fear of being sexually controlled. Although all three are closely connected, all three pains are different and need to be addressed individually in sexual healing.

### Second level of pain
The pain of submitting your sexual energy to one or both of your parents in the hope of receiving something else in return but not getting it. This can be seen in coming home from kindergarten or school with a painting you did and showing it to your parents in the hope of receiving the reward of love or congratulations, but not getting it.

### Third level of pain
The pain of being sexually controlled by one or both of your parents in order to receive love, which twists the subconscious statement of personal need in childhood from *I need sexual-energy connection in order to feel love* into the conscious statement of personal need in adulthood *I love having sexual-energy connection* or *I love having sex (in order to feel love)*. This does not imply that everyone who says *I love having sex* has a hidden unfulfilled need for parental love, but some people who say it do.

### Point 7: Kidney Meridians Running between the Navel and the Gracilis
The kidney meridians running between the navel and the uppermost medial side of the thigh house the characteristics of the sexual energies of your parents up to and including the act of your conception. The meridians are palpable between the navel and the top of the pubis, but then descend inward through the pelvic girdle to the inner tops of the thighs. These characteristics may be open and loving, causing warmth and softness in this area of the body, or these characteristics may be fearful, controlling, and loveless, causing cold and contraction in this area of the body. The section of kidney meridian running on the right hand side of your body houses the sexual energy of your father, while the section of meridian running on the left houses that of your mother.

## Point 8: The Navel

The navel is the portal through which the energy of the environment of your mother's womb enters your body. This energy extends from the center of the navel to various points in the pelvic girdle area, such as the hips, hamstrings, AIIS (anterior inferior iliac spine, or the anterior borders of the hip bones), and the groin. The quality of this environmental energy depends on the state of the health of your mother, her feelings about having you in her womb, and the environmental energy that she lived in while carrying you in her womb, including the energy of the relationship she was having with your father at the time. As with all forms of subtle-body energy, if the energy you lived in while you were in the womb was warm and loving, it would have created a similar warming, softening, opening, and trusting effect in your body. If, on the other hand, the energy was a bit cold or tight (maybe your parents were going through a bad patch during your stay in your mother's womb), then it would have created an environmental energy that would have had a similar cooling and tightening effect in your body, especially in the area around your navel. Generally speaking, in adulthood, the physiological effects of the energies you experienced in the womb are mild, unless something extreme happened while you were growing there.

# 5

# Spiritual Energy

The fifth and sixth chakras are the locations of spiritual energy in the body. The energies of these chakras are described as having such a high vibration as to lie outside the range of ordinary sense perception. Spiritual energy is an energy you cannot feel in the body of another person through the ordinary sense of touch. Instead, it passes through the body in the same way radio waves do. The way spiritual energy reveals its presence and development in the body is through the things you dream about or see in your meditations.

Dreams of being strangled, usually by a male character, and dreams of a male figure killing people are early signs that your spiritual centers are awakening. Such dreams symbolize the conscious mind, the ego, represented by the male dream character, reacting to the awakening of the higher-energy centers within your body. The higher-energy centers lead you to deep levels of truthful understanding about life. Indeed, one of the functions of the sixth chakra is to turn your understanding of life upside down, turning it on its head, or in the esoteric tradition, "As above, so below."

There is one part of you, however, that does not want you to reach this level of understanding. This is your conscious mind, the empirical, rational, logical part of you. This is the ego, always represented by a male character in dreams, which upon the awakening of the truth centers in

your body becomes threatened by such an awakening and so symbolically tries to stop the process by trying to strangle or kill it. A dream
of being strangled reveals the area of the body the ego is symbolically
trying to harm, the neck, which is in the area of the fifth chakra. This
reveals that the energy of the fifth chakra and the function of the fifth
chakra concerns truth—the revelation of truth, the freedom to speak
the truth, and the freedom to listen to the truth. The dream of the
male figure symbolically killing other people reveals the ego wanting to
symbolically kill the awakening of the higher-energy centers within you.
Both dreams reveal the same issue.

Dreaming of waterfalls and of seeing the faces of people you know
but who have died are additional signs that your spiritual energy has
awakened. Dreaming of dead people reveals a connection within you
between the three-dimensional world of space, location, and time, and
a world without physical form and physical definition. This connection
is spiritual energy, which bridges both dimensions. As energy, it is able
to pass through your physical body, bringing to you a fuzzy awareness
of a reality that lies outside your bodily awareness, outside your normal
sense-based reality. Spiritual energy can also be said to be the energy
that bridges the divide between the left hemisphere and the right hemisphere of the brain.

Spiritual energy is also the energy that causes you to wake up in the
middle of the night with a lightbulb moment of deep insight or intuitive understanding. It is the energy that causes you to wake up early in
the morning with an inspirational idea about how to improve your life
or your job.

If you are a student of yoga or massage who is also holding down a
day job, it is spiritual energy that will direct you to wake up one morning knowing what choice between the two to make. It is the moment
when your intellectually reasoned life choice is replaced by your intuitively directed life choice. Ironically, this is the moment your neck-
strangling ego wants to kill. It marks the stage in life where you begin
to listen to your intuition as well as to your intellect.

Intuition is the other great indicator of the presence of spiritual
energy within you. As a massage therapist, your sixth chakra, i.e., spiri-

tual energy, leads you to stop following the form and structure of the massage you have studied and to begin following an instinctive massage based on what your intuition tells you about the condition of your client when you touch them.

If a client comes to you for massage complaining of shoulder pain, it is your spiritual energy that will make you wonder if it is indeed your client's shoulder that is the cause of their discomfort, or if it is something deeper. Intellectual energy keeps you on the level of a rational understanding of your client's condition, so you will always treat your client at the point of their discomfort. Spiritual energy is the energy that gives you the ability to look deeper into the physical condition of your client to any hidden, underlying cause of their condition. Working with this level of insight, or spiritual wisdom, you can treat your massage client at both the point of manifestation and at the point of origin.

If you have ever given someone a massage wherein you suddenly lose all track of space and time, where you are so present in the massage that you lose all sense of your body and the body of your client and you lose sense of the space that separates you from your client, what you are experiencing is a manifestation of spiritual energy. It is the moment when you meet your client in a space that is both between you and yet, at the same time, contains both of you. It is the moment when you discover yourself in your client. It is when you experience the deep awareness that you are somehow part of that person and that the person is somehow part of you. It is when you realize that both you and your client are part of one extended being—that you and the other person are somehow one. This is the experience of universal oneness in the microcosm of oneness between therapist and client in massage. This is the moment when everything gets turned on its head ("As above, so below"), which is one of the functions of spiritual energy, for if your client is an extension of you and you are an extension of your client, then who exactly *is* your client? A separate being, or a projection of yourself?

Spiritual energy is the energy that transcends physical form, space, location, and time. It transcends intellectually based reality, sense-based perception, and physical boundaries. Spiritual energy, which reveals universal oneness, is the energy that transcends all forms of duality. This includes the duality of gender, too. This is very important in understanding the difference between spiritual energy and sexual energy, and in understanding that there is no connection between sexual energy and spiritual energy.

Spiritual energy does not recognize gender. Sexual energy, on the other hand, does. When trying to join together the internal male and female, you have to use an energy that transcends duality, not an energy that reinforces it. If you use sexual energy, which recognizes and reinforces the you/me, us/them duality, that energy is incapable of transcending this kind of duality. Therefore you cannot use sexual energy to connect to spiritual energy, an energy that does not recognize duality, an energy that is the expression of essential oneness. It is like trying to connect a space rocket with a semaphore; they are completely different states of being and comprise completely different energies.

## Awakening Spiritual Energy

Spiritual energy is joyously easy to awaken and develop. The way to do it is to align yourself to the functions of both the fifth and sixth chakras.

### The Fifth Chakra

The function of the fifth chakra is truth. The way to awaken your fifth chakra is to align yourself to the sources of the energy of truth. This can be as simple as listening to another person speaking his or her truth about a life experience. When you speak the truth, the energy that carries your spoken words to the ears of a listener is of a particular vibration, or frequency. This is the frequency of truth, the energy of truth. As a listener, when you listen to words of truth, the incoming energy of truth resonates with the hidden center of truth energy in yourself—the fifth chakra—awakening this energy center.

The same process occurs when you read a book that contains words of truth. When you read words of truth out loud, they generate the energy of truth. This energy then resonates within you, causing your own ability to discern the truth to awaken. The difficulty arises when you listen to someone who professes to speak the truth but doesn't, or when you read a book that purports to contain the truth but doesn't.

The great thing about the truth is that when shared, either through words, images, or symbols, it generates an energy that resonates at a particular frequency, which gives off a particular color: sky blue. The way to discern whether truth is being spoken or written or not is to bring the source to a shaman, spiritual healer, energy worker, or clairvoyant and ask whether the source is of the truth or not. If you are attracted to listening to a particular living guru or saint and you wish to know if that person is indeed a person of truth, get a photograph of that person. A photograph of a guru or a saint captures the invisible energy of that person. A shaman, spiritual worker, energy worker, or clairvoyant specializing in energy work will be able to discern the energy of that person from their photograph. If the person is a person of truth, there will be a particular energy, or color, to their photograph.

The same process applies to any book purporting to be a book of truth. The actual book, as a collection of printed words on pages of paper, will have a particular energy about it. Again, a shaman, spiritual healer, energy worker, or clairvoyant will be able to tell you whether the book does indeed contain the energy of truthfulness. Be aware that there are many sources of purported truth that are not (especially today!). The way to discern truth from untruthfulness is to check the energy of the source. Energy never lies. The energy of truth is always sky blue. The energy of untruth is yellow. You cannot fake this or conceal it.

## The Sixth Chakra

The function of the sixth chakra is to turn the rational, intellectual, empirical understanding of life on its head. It questions the nature of time, space, and location. It questions birth, life, and death. It questions everything we accept as real and offers the complete opposite as a legitimate alternative, a legitimate truth. For example, a traditional viewpoint of life is that God, or some powerful external force, created the world, whereas the spiritual viewpoint states that the world is a projection of your own mind and that you yourself are the creator.

The way to awaken the sixth chakra is to align yourself to a source of energy that has, or had, a fully awakened sixth chakra. These sources are usually acknowledged to be the great prophets or enlightened beings throughout history, such as Buddha. Aligning yourself to an enlightened being like Buddha is as easy as visiting a Buddhist temple and meditating, or sitting in front of an image of Buddha. This establishes a direct connection with the source, without an intermediary such as a priest or a monk or whatever. An image of Buddha is a symbol, a symbol that represents an energy of a very high vibration. By looking at such a symbol you will in time tune in to the energy of that symbol. This energy will then resonate in you and awaken a similar energy in yourself, awakening your sixth chakra, awakening your own inner Buddha.

Wherever possible, go straight to the source of enlightened energy. If your chosen symbol of enlightened energy is Jesus, then make a direct connection with Jesus. Visit a church and sit in front of a statue or image of him. Talk to him if you wish. Understand that the representation of Jesus is a symbol, and a symbol is a gateway to an energy that, when you connect to it, awakens a similar energy within yourself.

Symbols, whether words or images, are gateways to the awakening of the sixth chakra. The great thing about symbols is that they also reveal themselves in dreams and meditations. You don't always need books, statues, images, or guides. Although it can be greatly beneficial to have a living guide such as a priest, monk, or guru to help you understand the meaning of certain symbols, caution needs to be used when choosing a guide. Many symbols in spiritual texts are misinterpreted but are taught as being correct by living priests, monks, or gurus who are either innocently following a lineage of teaching that includes incorrectly interpreted symbols, or who have misinterpreted the symbols themselves. This is why it is important to discover the meanings of symbols yourself, through your own dreams and meditations.

The meaning of a symbol, whether in a spiritual text or in a series of dreams, changes as you evolve in your own spiritual development, and your understanding of it reflects where you are on your overall path toward understanding and enlightenment. If you listen to a guide who teaches only one meaning of a symbol, for example, the symbol of the loaves and the fishes, you become stuck in your spiritual development, as you are being held back by giving a symbol a fixed meaning instead of an evolving meaning. In this example, if you have chosen to follow Jesus as your source of spiritual nourishment, by asking him in prayer for loaves and fishes, you will receive many different interpretations over the years of your evolving relationship with him as your guide. If, on the other hand, you listen to a human guide who says that loaves and fishes represent nothing more than a historical reportage of sacks of food, then that part of your spiritual development will be blocked.

## What Spiritual Energy Feels Like

Spiritual energy is the energy that nourishes your spiritual understanding of life. Although it is energy, it is a very subtle form of energy, not robust enough to give you physical strength, nor robust enough to give rise to emotion. It does give rise to love, but a different kind of love than the emotional, heartfelt, or familial love experienced through direct physical connection with another person.

It is the energy that gives rise to inspiration and intuition. This is why spiritual energy has no tangible physiological or emotional component. It does, however, have a metaphysical feel to it. Spiritual energy makes you feel lighter. It can make you feel taller and less connected to the ground beneath your feet. In color it can be white, gold, sky blue, indigo, lilac, violet, ultraviolet, or purple. Metaphysically it is also an extremely hot energy.

It does, however, have one very interesting physiological characteristic: when spiritual energy visits you at night, you can sometimes feel it as a clear physical pressure being exerted on the top of your head. It is like someone pushing down on the top of your head with the palm of their hand. This lasts only a moment. The experience is usually associated with the spiritual energy referred to as "the all-seeing eye."

---

### The Experience of Working
### with Spiritual Energy in Yoga or Massage

When you teach yoga or you massage with spiritual energy, it enables you to convey great understanding or great healing in a very short space of time. Spiritual energy works at very high speed. After using or channeling spiritual energy, your body feels like it is the engine of a car that has been driven at 100 mph for two hours in third gear. This is why working with it can leave you temporarily exhausted afterward; it can cause your energy to short-circuit. You feel incredibly high, then you collapse, then you recover and rebalance, all within an hour or so. Most people cannot work with this energy for long periods of time. It needs to be counterbalanced with recovery and deep grounding.

---

## Spiritual Orgies

I am always amazed at how readily people will go into a room full of strangers and then, under the guidance of an appointed group leader, sit down, close their eyes, and begin to meditate and open their sixth chakras to the energies of the entire room. This is the same as going to an orgy and having sex with a roomful of strangers without care, without caution, and without proper protection. You have absolutely no idea what you could contract spiritually. It is the same as going into a roomful of financial investors, none of whom you know, laying your life savings out on the table and saying, "I am looking for a good investment." Some investors will genuinely want to help you, while others, if given half a chance, will take advantage of your innocence and fleece you of every penny you have.

When you open your sixth chakra, the third eye, you open up an energy center that is vulnerable to a type of energy that can be transmitted to you without the need for direct contact, whether direct physical contact, direct visual contact, or direct vocal contact. Sixth-chakra spiritual energy transcends all borders and boundaries, whether physical, such as the skeletal frame of your body, or mental, such as your determination to close your conscious mind off to external energies and ideas. There is a temptation to think that because you go to a group meditation, every person there must be good or decent because they too are doing meditation and not out drinking, partying, and being self-indulgent. Yes, there will be some good people in the room, but there may also be people with corrupted or misguided spiritual ideas looking to share them with others, for example, newcomers who are openly and innocently looking for answers or something to fill an inner feeling that something is missing, or leaders wanting to direct and control others.

The trouble is, people with corrupted or diseased spiritual energy do not have visible scabs or warts on their sixth chakra or puss oozing from their third eye by which we can identify them. They look no different from someone with clear, healthy spiritual wisdom. But given half a chance, they will fill you with spiritual "wisdom" that is not quite spiritual wisdom. Instead of being white light, it is tainted or dark in color. It won't have any adverse physical effect on you, but it will cause you to question or even reject true spiritual wisdom when it is subsequently offered to you. If it is your path to search for truth and move toward spiritual enlightenment, then what could cause you more illness than picking up spiritual energy that leads you off your path completely?

So, just as you risk contracting a sexually transmitted disease from enjoying a series of unprotected sexual encounters with a roomful of strangers at an orgy, you also risk contracting an STD when going to a group meditation and opening your sixth chakra to a roomful of strangers. STD, in this case, means *spiritually transmitted disease*. So practice safe spirit!

## The Myth of Achieving Enlightenment through Sex

Western countries have been influenced by many misleading teachers and gurus. There is a misconception that sex can lead to advanced spirituality, higher energy levels, and liberation. It has been suggested by some spiritual gurus—mostly males who want to have sex with young female disciples—that there is a direct connection between sexual energy and spiritual energy; in short, that sex with an enlightened person can lead an unenlightened person to liberation.

Connection is two-way. If sexual energy connects to spiritual energy, it follows that spiritual energy connects to sexual energy. In this way they are interconnected. In their interconnection, their energies flow between each other in both directions simultaneously. That is the nature of connection. If there were a direct connection between sexual energy and spiritual energy, it should be possible for a male spiritual guru to be able to bring his young female student to sexual orgasm through the practice of spiritual meditation. Bearing in mind that spiritual energy is an energy that transcends all forms of duality and time and space, and can pass through the physical body, the enlightened guru should theoretically be able to transmit his spiritual energy to his student without ever touching the person. And then, if spiritual energy has a connection to sexual energy, as this kind of guru says it does, he should be able to use his spiritual energy, transmitted to his student through meditation, to connect with the sexual energy of the student and thereby bring the person to sexual orgasm.

If you are considering having sex with your guru on the pretense that you and he think it will bring you spiritual awakening, ask him to first meditate you to orgasm. Tell him to sit in an adjoining room for the meditation. If he is unable or unwilling to bring you to orgasm, it reveals one or both of two things: 1) he has no true spiritual powers, and 2) there is no connection between spiritual energy and sexual energy.

If you have never experienced spiritual awakening but have experienced sexual orgasm, then at least you know what the outcome of the "meditate me to orgasm" experience should be: orgasm. If, on the other hand, you have had no experience of spiritual awakening, then you have no idea what the outcome of the "During deep meditation last night I was asked by my spiritual guides to offer my body to you so that, through my body, they can join with you and share in the blessed gift of spiritual awakening" experience should be. You are vulnerable to any explanation from your guru on the outcome of a sexual act you might have with him, even if that explanation is complete and utter rubbish.

The other thing to look out for in the spiritual guru who promises sexual awakening through sex is whether or not discrimination is a factor in your guru's invitation. Spiritual energy does not discriminate. This is because in spirit, where everything is one, there is nothing to discriminate between. There is no duality. There is no gender, no male and no female. True spiritual teaching does not preach discrimination. A true spiritual teacher like His Holiness the Dalai Lama does not discriminate in who comes to him for an audience. Everyone is welcome, regardless of age, gender, culture, nationality, or religion. If a spiritual guru professes to spread spiritual awakening through the act of sex, such a guru should be willing to do so without discriminating based on gender. He should have sex with men as well as with women, unattractive people as well as beautiful people, older people as well as younger people. To use a sports metaphor, the guru should also be catching as well as pitching. If what this guru says is true, he should be having sex with as many people as possible, without consideration as to gender, age, or appearance, as this would help spread spiritual awakening more quickly and to a wider audience. Yet most male spiritual gurus who profess a desire to spread spiritual awakening through sex tend to have sex with young, attractive females only. This is an expression of preference. And any guru expressing preference in bringing about enlightenment in a person is not expressing true spirituality or true enlightenment.

People trained in sound healing frequently use Tibetan bowls, tuned to resonate at different frequencies, to awaken and cleanse the energies of the different chakras. The healing bowl tuned to resonate at the energy frequency of the second chakra, the sexual chakra, vibrates at a different frequency than the healing bowl tuned to resonate to the energy frequency of the sixth chakra, which houses spiritual energy. The second chakra resonates at 210 Hz, whereas the sixth chakra resonates at 221Hz. If you program 210 Hz into an audio oscillator and play the signal through an amplifier and speaker, you will hear a sound wave with a frequency of 210 Hz. Even when you increase the volume, the frequency of the sound remains at 210 Hz. No matter what you do, you cannot turn the 210-Hz sound wave into a 221-Hz sound wave. The same principle applies to the energy of the chakras. No matter how much you ram the 210-Hz sexual energy of your second chakra into the energy system of another person, it cannot produce 221-Hz sixth-chakra spiritual energy. They are energies of a completely different frequency and have no connection whatsoever. One is orange, the other indigo.

## The Relationship between Sexual Energy and Spiritual Energy

Though there is not a direct connection between sexual energy and spiritual energy in the sense that sexual energy cannot be transmuted into spiritual energy, there is a notable relationship between the second chakra and the sixth. Recall from our discussion in chapter 2 that each chakra contains the resonant colors of all the other chakras. The stimulation of second-chakra energy through the act of sex activates the layer of second-chakra energy within both the first and sixth chakras. As the function of the first chakra is to reconnect to God, and the function of the sixth chakra is to transcend the reality of the three-dimensional world, two of the resulting feelings from sex can be a feeling of being closer to God and a feeling of transcending this three-dimensional reality. These are more commonly experienced among people with strongly open first or sixth chakras. This kind of sexual experience is sometimes misinterpreted as being deeply spiritual. Although intensely pleasurable, these types of experiences are not spiritual in nature, they are sense-based phenomena that expand your normal range of "feels-like" experience. Spiritual energy has no such associated feeling or experience, as it lies outside the realm of sense-based perception.

Such spiritual feelings following sex last as long as the layers of second-chakra energy within the first or sixth chakras remain stimulated. As soon as the energy in the second-chakra layer within the first and sixth chakras returns to its normal state, the feelings of closeness to God or dimensional transcendence dissipate. Depending on the intensity and duration of the stimulation of the second-chakra layer in the first and sixth chakras, the feelings of spiritual awakening can continue well after the second-chakra layers have been activated and stimulated. But note that no direct connection between the orange layer in the sixth chakra and the indigo layer in the sixth chakra has been made. As previously stated, they are energies of different frequencies and cannot activate each other. Spiritual awakening is spiritual awakening. Once it is awakened, it remains awake. If any spiritual feelings dissipate following an act of sex, then no awakening has taken place.

### A Detailed Explanation of the Aforementioned

Let's recall our discussion of the anatomy of a chakra in chapter 2. A chakra consists of seven layers of energy of different vibrations and frequencies circling a central core, which is an energy of yet another, different frequency. Each of the seven layers gives off a governing color corresponding to its particular frequency. These colors are easily seen by shamans, clairvoyants, energy workers, and spiritual healers trained in energy work or who are sensitive to the color of energy. The colors, from the lower to the higher chakras, are: red, orange, yellow, green, sky blue, indigo, and purple. In each chakra, purple is the color found closest to the central core of a chakra, as seen in figure 5.1 below. Red is the color found furthest from the central core. The central core of a chakra consists of an energy that gives off a brilliant white color.

We know the human body has seven major chakras. The brilliant white light at the core of each of the major chakras is a powerful form of energy that appears in all dimensions and universes and is felt by many

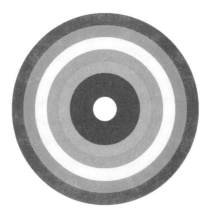

*Fig. 5.1. The second chakra in a state of balance before sex
(remember that each individual chakra contains
all seven layers of color around a white core).*

to be the energy that represents oneness, unlimitedness, and transcendence. We also use other terms, such as *the Tao, Atman, God, Buddha,* or *enlightenment,* to refer to this source energy. Although each chakra contains energy of seven different colors, or frequencies, each individual chakra has an overall characteristic color that is based on the function and purpose of the particular chakra.

The chakras are connected. The brilliant white core in the first chakra is connected to the brilliant white core in the second chakra, which is connected to the brilliant white core in the third chakra, and so on up to the seventh chakra. The connection between the central cores of brilliant white light in each of the chakras runs along the spinal cord up to the brain stem, along the sushumna nadi. Similarly, the layers of red energy in each of the chakras are connected, as are the orange layers in each chakra, the yellow layers, and the green, sky blue, indigo, and purple layers, with each color connected to the same color in all the other chakras. Although the connection between the central cores of brilliant white light in the seven chakras runs through the sushumna nadi, or along the spinal cord, the connections between the other layers of colored energy in the chakras do not run through the sushumna channel. Sexual energy does not run along the spinal cord.

During sex, the orange layer in the second chakra, which is associated with sexual energy, becomes greatly stimulated and expands beyond the second chakra, connecting to the layers of orange energy in all the other chakras in the body, thus expanding the range of feeling and pleasure experienced throughout the body (see figure 5.2). The other layers of energy in each of the chakras, including the layers of indigo energy, remain unaffected. Upon entering the first chakra, the overstimulated orange energy from the second chakra triggers the layer of orange energy in the first chakra, triggering feelings related to one or some of the functions of the first chakra. Two of the main functions of the first chakra are connection to God, and, in the absence of God, connection to family. This is why during sex people with strongly developed and open first chakras can often feel closer to God and may even feel like conceiving a child. Upon experiencing this feeling, it's not uncommon to hear the person exclaim, "Oh God!"

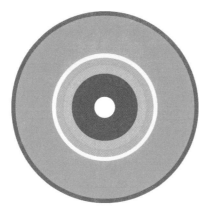

*Fig. 5.2. The second chakra during sex:*
*the layer of orange energy becomes greatly stimulated.*

As the flow of stimulated orange energy rises upward through the chakras, it enters the fourth chakra, where it triggers feelings of love. Upon experiencing this feeling, many people in the middle of sex blurt out, "I love you."

Upon entering the fifth chakra, stimulated orange energy triggers feelings of truthfulness. Upon experiencing these feelings, many people in the middle of sex feel like saying something truthful like, "This is the happiest I have ever been."

Upon entering the sixth chakra, the stimulated energy of the orange layer triggers feelings of transcending time and space. Upon experiencing these feelings, some people try to express this as some sort of transdimensional state or alternative universe, where everything feels connected, or is one.

So yes, the sixth chakra does become activated during sex, but only in the orange layer, the energy governing feeling, pleasure, and sense-based perception. The spiritual energy of the sixth chakra, housed in the indigo layer, is unaffected. This is also why, following sex, the levels of feeling and pleasure fade, and no lasting spiritual state remains.

### Out-of-Body Experiences during Sex

Some people regularly have out-of-body experiences during sex. This is a sign of imbalance in the second chakra. Maybe something traumatic happened to this person in their early childhood that caused it to be painful to be fully present in their body at that time. To escape the pain, they began to create and live in the world of their mind instead, anything to get away from the pain of the physical environment they were in. They found more peace in their mind than in their body. Now in adulthood, during sex, when the second chakra, which is associated with early childhood, is stimulated, they automatically leave their body, which is a default reaction. All that is happening is that a pattern of behavior that was established during an earlier time in life, the period governed by the second chakra, is being triggered through the act of sex. The person might find such an out-of-body experience to be pleasurable and intense, but it is not exactly a spiritual experience. It is an escape from the body, an act of defense and protection against an old hurt being triggered.

# 6

# Interpersonal, Ancestral, and Environmental Energies

Between you and certain people and environments in your life exist energetic connections that bind you to that person, group, or situation. That's why it is sometimes difficult to let go of someone or something from your past. Even when you do not see a person anymore, the energetic connection you had with him or her and the effects of that energetic connection remain. The same can apply to certain groups you were a part of or other aspects of your life in the past.

## Interpersonal Connections

The effects of the energetic connection you have with a person depend on three factors: 1) the type of person you connect with; 2) the depth or strength of that connection; and 3) the duration of that connection. Some energetic connections you experience with a person are very light and not lasting. For example, you meet someone new in a social situation and discover, through conversation, that you have a shared passion, and through further conversation you share your passion and energy for that particular subject. You are happy to talk, and your new friend is happy to listen. As well, your new friend is happy to talk, and you are happy to listen. This is a very basic form of exchange between two people, resulting in a temporary energy exchange or connection. After the social event, however, you will probably never see that person again. In time you may forget that you ever met them. There is no connection remaining. This type of energetic connection has no lasting effect on you.

The energetic connection two people make in a casual social situation runs between the third chakras of both parties. The color of the energy connection is therefore yellow. There is no sexual connection, the energy of which belongs to the second chakra. There is no familial connection, the energy of which belongs to the first chakra. There is no love connection, the energy of which belongs to the fourth chakra.

Third-chakra connections not only apply to people you meet in social situations, they also apply to most of the people you encounter at work, including colleagues, employers, and employees, and the people you encounter in any learning environment, whether fellow students, teachers, or your own students (if you are a teacher). The energy that comes through such a contact enters your body through your third chakra and is then distributed throughout your body along the energy channels, or meridians, associated with the third chakra—the spleen, stomach, liver, and gallbladder meridians, as delineated by TCM. When the energy of connection that is coming into you through your third chakra is open, warm, free, positive, supportive, and encouraging, as in the quality of energy that comes from a good teacher or an encouraging employer, there are resulting positive effects felt throughout the area of your third chakra and the areas ruled by the spleen, stomach, liver, and gallbladder meridians.

Not all teachers, employers, or colleagues are so free and encouraging in their energetic connection with you, however. Some may try to use the energy of control with you, while others may try to generate fear in you. Such connections will result in tightness or coldness in your solar plexus. This cold or tightening energy is then carried throughout your body on the stomach-spleen and liver-gallbladder meridians, adversely effecting body areas associated with these meridians, such as the shoulder area around the trapezius, the sides of the neck, the sides of the jaws, and the upper digestive system. Although you may feel the effects of workplace stress in your shoulders, jaws, and digestive system, it is useful to know that the energy that is causing this distress is entering your body through your solar plexus, your third chakra. Therefore, when seeking treatment for stress, it is helpful to find a bodyworker or massage therapist specializing in energy work, who can work on your third chakra to release you from the energy of stress at its source. This work can be further supported by additional energy work on the corresponding meridians that distribute the energy of stress around your body. This is usually a very effective treatment for stress.

## Energetic Connections in Intimate Relationships

The energetic connection you have with someone you meet in a social situation changes completely if you commence a sexual relationship with that person. Although the physical connection is through the sexual organs, the energetic connection is between the second chakras of both persons. Sexual energy entering your body through your second chakra is distributed around your body on the energy channel, or meridian, associated with the second chakra: the kidney meridian. Some sexual connections are warm, fun, happy, playful, curious, sensuous, and exciting. The connection is given and received freely, and is not governed by rules, expectations, or hidden, unfulfilled needs. When shared freely, such sexual energy exchanges leave no lingering adverse effects.

Sexual encounters can sometimes develop into more long-term, complex relationships. In such a case the range of energetic connections expands. People can move in together and share possessions and finances. This is a sharing of third-chakra energy, connecting both people energetically in the area of the solar plexus. Often people fall in love, developing a fourth-chakra heart-energy connection. While building trust and openness in the relationship, each person may begin to reveal their inner selves to their partner, developing a connection in the energy center that governs the truth, the fifth chakra. Some couples may even develop a mutual interest in spiritual matters, developing a connection in the energy center relating to spiritual development, the sixth chakra. Thus it is possible to be in a relationship with another person and be connected energetically with that person through your second, third, fourth, fifth, and sixth chakras.

That is why when such a relationship breaks down, it can be very difficult to sever all the different energetic connections. Yet any energy connection can be undone. The process must be two-way, however. You cannot let go of someone who is not ready to let go of you. If there is someone you need to let go of, such as a former lover, boyfriend, or girlfriend, but you are finding it impossible to do so, you need to understand that you have an energetic connection to that person, and then work with a trained shaman, energy worker, or spiritual healer to determine what type of energy connection you have with the person. This may reveal any hidden, subconscious needs you may have of that person that need to be acknowledged and understood. Understand too that the other person is similarly connected to you energetically. With the same shaman or energy worker, you can determine the nature of the energy that connects your significant other to you, to determine any hidden, subconscious needs they have of you. Note that the other person does not need to be present for this process.

The reason why it is important to reveal any subconscious needs existing between you and your ex-partner is that it is almost always the energies of unfulfilled, hidden, subconscious needs that continue to bind you to the person you are trying to break free of, and vice versa. For instance, a former partner may admit that the reason he was with you was because you were good-looking and the sex was great, whereas behind this excuse he really needed to be with you because of the feeling of security he got from you. This was his subconscious need of you, and not understanding this can be the reason why you never felt that the relationship added up, or why he is more upset than you expected upon breaking up. He is unwilling to let you go because his ongoing, subconscious need for security is very strong.

Once you fully understand the nature of the connection you had with that person, including any hidden, subconscious needs, you are in a position to be able to forgive him, especially if he caused you pain. Once you can forgive, you can let go completely. At the same time, through the honest investigation of the energies that connected you with your ex-partner, you give him a similar opportunity to forgive you and let you go.

---

### Breaking Free from the Energy Connection of Your Last Relationship

This is a nice little exercise I learned from my energy teacher in Chiang Mai, Jasmine Vishnu, at a time when I was experiencing a pattern of hurtful relationships. The exercise is designed to help break the connections from your last relationship. You can do this exercise without your ex-partner being present. Although you can try this exercise by yourself, it is advised that you use a guide or teacher the first time you try it, if possible. A guide can help make sure you are open and grounded, and that a proper connection has been established between you and your ex-partner. Begin as follows:

Open all your energy centers and ground yourself deeply.

Summon up an image of your last partner.

Stand them in front of you, and while looking directly into their eyes . . .

Blow back what you saw of them through your eyes.

Blow back what you thought of them with your voice.

Blow back how your heart felt about them through your heart.

Blow back their sexual energy from your second chakra.

Let them "feel" the consequences of their returned energies. See if they make any facial gestures, then wait for them to speak.

If they say something, answer truthfully, only truthfully. No accusations. Do not accuse them of being a bitch or a little shit.

Tell them how you feel. Tell them how they made you feel. Speak your truth at all times.

Let them speak freely in return. No accusation, no judgment, no interruption.

When you have found a comfortable amount of peace in the exercise, you can stop.

You will be amazed by what the other person says to you in the final step of this exercise. The great advantage of having a higher-consciousness communication with someone who is not present is that they never lie in their answers to your questions. Higher-consciousness communication is incapable of lying.

## Breaking Free from a Pattern of Hurtful Relationships

You may realize that the hurtful dynamics in your last relationship are part of an ongoing pattern that has run through all your intimate relationships, and you want to break this pattern. To do so, start with the exercise outlined above, beginning with the person who hurt you in your most recent relationship. When you have found a comfortable amount of peace with that person, move on to the next-to-last hurtful relationship, and so on, until you find the relationship you had when you first let someone hurt, manipulate, control, or betray you. Upon uncovering that relationship and resolving it, the pattern of suffering from hurtful relationships is largely broken. Note that to break the pattern completely, you have to thoroughly investigate your early relationship with your opposite-sex parent.

I have personal experience with this exercise, and it subsequently changed the kind of person who became attracted to me. The old pattern in my relationships that I had to uncover and understand was that of "I give of myself without standing up for myself when I receive nothing in return." In relationship situations this repeatedly attracted to me people who knew they could take from me without my getting upset with them when they gave nothing in return. This was the energetic pattern in my relationships, a pattern certain people were able to subconsciously sense in me.

Upon breaking this pattern, I no longer attracted women who were happy to take from me without giving anything in return. This initially led to a short period of confusion for me, as *I* was still attracted to the same type of woman, the woman who took from me, but that type of woman was no longer attracted to me because I had broken the pattern of allowing partners to take from me without giving in return. I had to quickly relearn about adult relationships. Before I broke the pattern, I was used to being treated badly in my relationships, indeed being treated badly was my proof that I was in a relationship. When I was being treated well, I was unable to trust the relationship. It took about a year to settle into the new pattern of being treated well. Once broken, however, moving from the old pattern of attraction to the new one happened immediately.

## Familial Connections

The energetic connections that bind you to the members of your family, your parents in particular, are among the most difficult to understand and unravel. These kinds of connections also have the greatest range of effects on your physical body. To understand why you sometimes feel coldness, contraction, tightness, or pain in certain areas of your body, sometimes it is necessary to look beyond your immediate circumstances to what was passed on to you at the time of your conception.

### *Energy Connections between You and Your Parents—Ancestral Energy*

We carry second-generation energetic imprints of both our father and our mother from the time of our conception, as described in the discussion of sexual energy in chapter 4. To recapitulate: the energy your father used to conceive you contains a microcosm of all the energies of his entire life, from the time of his own birth to the time of your conception, including his own experiences of life, his beliefs, his behaviors, and his emotional experience of life. So if, for example, your father experienced a lonely childhood, and the unacknowledged and unreleased energy of that childhood loneliness was housed in his sit bones, a second-generation copy of this energy will be mapped onto your own body in the very same place, and as a result you will carry your father's unreleased pain in your own sit bones. If you experienced a warm and loving start in life, then this warm energy will help dissolve the cold energy of your father's lonely childhood from your sit bones, thus leaving behind no adverse physical effects. If, on the other hand, you too experienced a cold, loveless, and otherwise difficult start in life, this cold energy mixes with the cold energy of your father's cold start in life, exaggerating the condition in your sit bones. This cold energy leads to contraction in the hamstrings, more commonly known as tight hamstrings.

The same applies to your mother. She too passed on a copy of the totality of her life-experience energy to you at the time of your conception. This energy can have a similar warming or cooling effect in certain parts of your body, based on where that energy was imprinted in her body. This is how ancestral energy works between parents and children—you too will pass along an energetic imprint of your own makeup to your own children if you have children. This is the energetic web that links one generation to another, all the way back through one's ancestral line.

### The Energy of Your Early Environment

The organ through which you receive the energy of your earliest environment, the womb of your mother, is the umbilical cord. The umbilicus is attached to the navel. The incoming energy of your environment enters your body through your navel and from there extends to various points in your pelvic girdle, including your hips, groin, AIIS (anterior border of the hip bones), and the tops of hamstrings. It also runs between the navel and the top of the pubic bone along the kidney meridian and on the back of the body between L3 and L5 along the urinary bladder meridian. Generally speaking, the physiological effects of the environmental energies of the womb are mild unless something extreme happens, for example, your father leaving your mother halfway through the time she was pregnant with you.

After your birth, a new energy connection develops between you and your parents. This is the connection you have with the energy of your postbirth external environment, the energy of your home, the energies that exist between you and your mother and father, and the energy that exists between your parents. This postbirth environmental energy enters your body through the root chakra, at the base of your torso, in your perineum. From the perineum, this energy travels through your pelvic girdle upward into your lower abdomen, to a level roughly midway between your navel and the top of your pubic bone. If the energy of your earliest home environment was cold, the energy in this area of your body will be similarly cold, with contraction of the tissues, organs, muscles, and blood vessels there. If there was a cold relationship between you and your parents in your early years, you will feel a coldness of energy in the area between your pubic bone and the midpoint between your navel and the top of your pubic bone. If the coldness existed between you and your mother, the coldness will be to the left of this area; it will be to the right if the coldness was between you and your father.

In this discussion of the energetic connections that exist between parents and children, it's worth reiterating that whatever energetic imprints we have received from our parents we will pass along to our own children. I am unable to report on this connection personally, as I have no children of my own. However, I once asked a good friend of mine who is a mother where she feels her connection to her children is, and she replied: in her sacrum.

---

### The Inability to Tell the Difference between Your Energy and the Energy of Others

Awareness of your own identity is a function of the first chakra. A strong first chakra gives the feeling: This is who I am. I know who I am. I am happy being in my own skin and body. The ability to tell the difference between what is yours and what is someone else's comes after this first-chakra foundation of self-identity and is a function of the second chakra. The inability to tell the difference between your energy and the energy of your massage clients or yoga students reveals an imbalance in your first and second chakras.

At its root, this imbalance is an imbalance between what is yours and what is your parents'. If in earliest childhood you were not given sufficient energy of recognition, love, and reward, you were left with insufficient energy necessary to develop your first chakra. The result is a first chakra lacking in any sense of who it is, unable to clearly state: This is me. I own me. I am responsible for me. I make my own decisions. Yet it is full of the energy of your early environment—your parents and the things in their lives that got in the way of their giving you sufficient recognition, love, and rewards necessary for your own development. In this regard you have grown up with a lesser awareness of yourself but a greater awareness of your environment and your parents. You identify more with your environment and with your parents than you do with yourself. As a result, in adulthood you find yourself more aware of and sensitive to the feelings and emotions of others than you are of your own feelings and emotions.

This scenario actually makes for the ideal healer or therapist. You can easily tune in and read your client. While this sounds positive, it has its downside. You may find yourself easily taking on the energy of your client, while at the same time finding it difficult to protect yourself. You take on the identity of your client, as your own identity has not been strongly enough established to be self-standing and independent. This is a reenactment of what happened between you and your parents in your earliest childhood. In infancy, if you were unable to defend or protect yourself against the energies of your parents, especially if they were hurtful energies, you will find in adulthood that you are similarly unable to protect or defend yourself fully from the hurtful energies found in the bodies of some massage clients.

Massage or healing makes for an easy career fit for adults who, in their childhood, were not given sufficient energy to develop their own sense of self. Their sense of self was determined heavily by the needs of parents, whom they continually had to serve or make happy in order to protect themselves against potential pain or hurt. This is the adult who in childhood was trained to serve the needs of others. In serving others, they find their sense of self. This is the adult who is "happy" to help others, but the happiness they have in serving others is born out of the fear of being hurt if they do not serve them or make them happy. This is a hurtful pattern of behavior to be trapped in and sadly is a common pattern among those who practice massage and energetic healing. It is also the root of emotional burnout in massage, when the therapist who gives in order to receive does not receive what they subconsciously need.

The good news is that it is possible to break the pattern of not being able to tell the difference between your energy and the energy of your students or clients or others in your life. The energies that form and hold this pattern lie in the first chakra. If it was your mother who exerted the greater adverse effect in your infancy, the area of this energy will be more to the left side of the first-chakra area; if it was your father, it will be more to the right side of this area. If you hold this pattern, the energy in these areas of your body will be cold. The cold energy causes a freezing and contraction of the muscles, nerves, blood vessels, and organs in these areas of the body. It also causes strong contraction in the energy meridians running through these areas, which additionally blocks the flow of subtle-body energy through your groin and upper legs. This whole area of your body may be diagnosed as being blocked or empty of energy.

Consult with a shaman, energy worker, or spiritual healer trained in first-chakra healing and ask them to help you work through the energies and issues housed in this area of the body. Yoga, of course, is a wonderfully healing therapy for the first chakra. The healing process of yoga, however, is designed to unfold naturally and slowly, and it will take a longer period of time to work its magic than the time it would take a trained energy healer.

Once you have worked to release the energies of your early childhood environment that blocked the development of your self-identity, you will have the space to start growing the energy of self-identity. Once a strong sense of self has been built back into the first chakra, then the energy you use to differentiate your energy from that of your client, which is housed in the second chakra, will flow the way it should.

Some massage therapists, initially unable to tell the difference between their energy and the energy of their client, find that in time they become able to tell the difference. This happens when they become successful in their massage, adding to their confidence and strengthening their self-identity. With a strengthening sense of self-identity, they become more aware of their own energy, and with this growing sense of their own energy, they begin to recognize energy that is not their own. It is a beautiful example of using your massage or yoga practice to heal yourself.

## Breaking Energetic Connections with Your Parents

How you approach this depends on your personal philosophy and preferences. Some adults are not aware they have energetic connections to their parents. If they are happy in life, then they have no need to go looking for something they are not aware of, that is seemingly not causing any problems. Why should they? Then again some people do not accept that an energetic connection between themselves and their parents even exists, and they do not support energy work and the healing of energy in general. They accept that there is a connection, just not an energetic one. Then there are those people whose hearts are open, strong, and free enough to completely forgive their parents for any hurtful event that might have occurred with one or both parents. This level of forgiveness sets a person free of all energetic connections. This is unconditional forgiveness. Forgiving without needing to know what you are forgiving.

Those who have been properly trained in the arts of energetic or spiritual healing are capable of sending to the light any energies of previous hurtful experiences between parents and children. By sending the energy of hurt to the light, it is dissolved. Some exceptional healers are able to remove the energy of hurt in the body of a person through prayer, incantation, or chanting. Some people, trained in psychotherapy, counsel a full understanding of any hurtful events that occurred between a person and their parents, and from that point of understanding can help free the person from old pain, allowing them to move forward. As well, some forms of meditation train you to allow the energy of hurtful connections to release from within your body and to pass through your levels of awareness, including your memory and emotions, while not reacting to them. This starves the conscious mind of the way it wants you to react, so that in time your conscious mind gives up trying to get you to react. In this way you end up breaking free of the cycle of pain.

In certain instances of spiritual communication, such as those with Ascended Masters conducted through a trained medium, you can be counseled to let go of everything—to let go of all hurt, current and previous, remembered and not remembered. In one such instance I was guided by the Ascended Master Kuthumi: "It is not necessary to understand it. Let it go. Feel the unease and accept it." I have found this to be true in my own deep spiritual meditation. Spirit is not interested in whatever hurt you have suffered in life. It only wants you to let go of everything. This spiritual advice flies in the face of the conscious mind's understanding of forgiveness, which is that the original hurt must be brought into the light of conscious awareness so that we know what we are forgiving. As discussed in chapter 2, one of the functions of spiritual energy is to turn our conscious-mind understanding of life on its head.

Some teachers, such as my own, counsel that you investigate any pain you have in your body until it self-reveals its origin. Further investigation of the origin of the pain unveils a full understanding behind the circumstances of the original event, which then puts you in a position to let go of everything. For example, if you have a pain in your body that is related to the experience of being unloved in childhood, you fully investigate that pain until it leads you to the deepest point of being unloved, and then through that point to reveal the truth behind why you were unloved. You end up with the understanding that you were never meant to be unloved; certain circumstances just got in the way of your parents showing their love for you. When you then feel you were meant to be loved, you are free to reconnect to that love and to feel that you have always been loved, even though your life experience was the opposite. When you reconnect to the love that was once blocked, then the pain of the energy of being unloved is set free.

If it is your choice to self-investigate the energy of pain in your body that you sense comes from the relationship you had with your parents, be aware that you may need to investigate up to three types of energy: 1) the energy of your childhood environment; 2) the energy of your mother's womb; and 3) the energies of your parents' lives. Your parents don't have to be alive for you to do this investigation. A properly trained energy worker, spiritual healer, or shaman can help you connect with the consciousness or spirit of whomever has passed, enabling you to get a full understanding of their life, including any aspects that have been hidden from you and are subconsciously causing hurt in your body. There is no guarantee you will break all the hurtful connections you may have had with your parents, but you will be able to break most of them, regardless of which path of healing you take.

## The Energetic Connection between You and Your Siblings

There is a saying: *to be joined at the hip.* It refers to people who are so close, doing everything together, that they appear to have an actual physical bond. This saying points to the physical location of the energetic connection that exists between you and your siblings, or, for that matter, your spouse: the hips. Specifically, the energetic connection between you and your brother (or husband) is at the outside tip of the right-side iliac crest. The energetic connection between you and your sister (or wife) is at the outside edge of the left-side iliac crest.

As it always is with subtle energy, when the nature of the energy in this connection is warm, the parallel physiological effect in the corresponding part of the body is warming, strengthening, and opening. But if, for example, there is a painful connection between you and your brother, in energy work it will show up as an area of black energy on the otherwise red energy of the right iliac crest. Black, in this instance, reveals the presence of the energy of pain. If this is the case, there will be a corresponding pain in the outside edge of your right iliac crest. This black energy of pain sometimes trickles down the outside of the leg, causing pain in the leg and making walking difficult. A properly trained energy healer will be able to pull this black energy out of your iliac crest, resulting in a temporary freedom from this pain. I say "temporary" because for most people with a painful connection to either a sibling or a spouse, they must, at some stage, return to that sibling or spouse, and when that happens, the painful connection is reestablished.

## Recognizing Yourself in Your Massage Client

It is not unusual as a massage therapist to find you have some clients who are more difficult to deal with than others—not because they suffer from a difficult or complex condition, but because it is not easy to open yourself to them. You may experience some kind of resistance to working with them, or you may find yourself agitated when working with them. If you are honest with yourself, you may admit that you are afraid of working with them. At the end of a treatment you may find yourself feeling unwell. The novice massage therapist is tempted to say that the reason for feeling unwell after such a massage is that they have taken on the "bad energy" of that client. There is a temptation to blame the client. Although this sounds like a legitimate explanation, it is usually mistaken.

Clients are either male or female. The degree of openness and comfort you enjoy with your clients is at all times a perfect mirror of the degree of openness and comfort you enjoy with partners, spouse, and, most important, with your family. Furthermore, the type of relationship you have had with your parents is the yardstick that will establish the kind of relationships you have with your massage clients. If you have had an open and loving relationship with both your parents, you will have similar open and loving connections with both genders of your massage clients. There will be no feelings of resistance, agitation, fear, or illness with any of your massage clients. By extension, your clients will feel your love and openness and will be happy to receive from you over and over again.

Not everyone has such open and loving relationships with their parents and other family members and it is the degree of resistance and fearfulness that you have experienced with your parents or others in your family that is mirrored by the resistances and unease you experience with certain massage clients. If, for instance, you are a female therapist who has suffered from a harmful relationship with your father, with whom you are no longer open and whom you have not forgiven for what he did to you, it will be impossible for you to be honestly open and receptive to certain massage clients. There are three types of clients you will experience difficulties with or who will make you feel unwell after massaging: 1) the male client who has badly treated his daughter; 2) the male client whose pain is related to his feelings of guilt and his need for forgiveness for the way he badly treated his daughter; and 3) the female client whose pain is related to low self-esteem because of the way she was badly treated by her father (mirroring your own lack of self-love as a result of the way you were treated by your father).

As a therapist, you do not normally talk about family history with a new client, nor would you have questions relating to family history on your intake form, and, of course, a new client will be very unwilling to disclose their family history, especially if some form of abuse was involved. All you know is that your client is experiencing physical discomfort and that they are coming to you for treatment for their pain. What you do not know, at this early stage, is that their pain is related to family history. When you treat this client and touch their pain, you will inexplicably feel some degree of illness yourself. This because through your massage you have touched on unresolved pain relating to your own personal history.

There is enormous benefit in working with a client who makes you feel unwell in this way. The temptation is to stop working with such a person, or to take forms of protection to keep you from feeling unwell while working with them. But the real opportunity in working through such a situation comes from asking yourself: Why do I feel this way when I work with this person? What is it about this person that makes me feel unwell or uneasy? The client who makes you feel ill during or after treatment represents an opportunity to examine yourself and your life and to face your own hidden pain. If treating a male client makes you angry, is it because you are angry with your client, or is it maybe because you still hold within yourself a lot of unreleased or unrecognized anger toward your father?

The secret healing that happens in massage is when you use your massage client as a mirror, as a means to diagnose yourself. When you form your self-diagnosis, you have the opportunity to work on yourself and heal yourself of your pain by bringing your truth into the light of conscious awareness. In this example, when you have fully let go of any anger you may have relating to your father, you will find that you will never again experience anger with a male client in your massage practice. This is self-healing in massage: recognize yourself in your massage client. Heal yourself of the pains your client mirrors in you. As you begin healing yourself of all your life pains, you automatically begin healing all your clients of the same life pains.

## Aligning with the Energy of a Yoga or Massage System or Teacher

As a yoga practitioner, you are probably following a particular system of yoga, practicing and attending the classes of a teacher (or teachers) within that system at his or her yoga studio. What you may not realize is that the system of yoga you practice was developed by an individual with a specific intention in personal achievement through that system and that the studio in which you practice was set up by a person with a specific goal in mind—in other words, that your teacher is teaching with a specific intention of achieving something personally from their practice of teaching within that system.

Developing a system of yoga or setting up a yoga studio starts with a need on the part of the person who starts it. This could be the need to achieve something, such as building up a successful business. Or it could be the need to fulfill something, such as an unfulfilled childhood need to be taken seriously. Or it might be the need to share something, such as a beloved lineage of yoga. Whatever the need or needs, it becomes the founding energy of the yoga studio, whose purpose is to fulfill that need. This becomes the founding energy of the yoga you practice and the environment in which it is practiced. Make no mistake, it is there to fulfill the energetic needs of its creator or founder.

Let's say someone develops a strong, dynamic, physical form of yoga because they need a yoga that helps them dissipate energies and tensions they have in their body, which they are unable to release naturally through being grounded, or which they are unable to release through other, less dynamic, more yin systems of yoga or bodywork. They therefore develop a system of yoga through which they can dissipate inner tension. This is the founding energy with which that system of yoga was developed: the need to dissipate and release through a strong, dynamic practice.

This form of yoga is then developed and taught to others. Regardless of the mechanics of the practice, the form of yoga will best suit those who also need a yoga practice through which they can dissipate tension and feel more grounded. This is where the needs of the student are in alignment with the founding energy of the yoga studio: the need to dissipate and ground. A student who is already naturally grounded might be attracted to this system of yoga due to the overall form and sequence of asanas, yet their need to practice yoga is not to dissipate energy and ground themselves, something they can already do. Such a student will indeed enjoy this particular yoga practice but will not receive the full benefit of the practice, as their true need for yoga is not in alignment with the needs this approach to yoga was developed to fulfill.

### What You Don't Know May Hurt You

The way to receive the full benefit of a yoga system is to find the studio whose original founding needs are in alignment with your own needs for practice. An attractive-looking yoga studio may look like the one you want, but if its founding energy is not in alignment with your needs, you will not receive its full benefit. You may find that after several months, or even several years, of practice, it is not the yoga for you.

Then too, in some yoga studios there is a hidden agenda, a need of you, as a student, that is never advertised or discussed. This is why you can sometimes enter the premises of a yoga studio and intuitively know it is not right for you. That's because yoga studios trade on energy, most commonly the energy of teaching in return for the energy of money. This trade is openly advertised in the form of a fee per class. This is an open, clear contract, and once agreed to by both parties, it creates no problems. However, conflicts occur when a yoga studio needs something more from you that they do not openly advertise: specifically, they need you for your energy. They actually need you more for your energy than for your money.

Let's go back to our original premise. Most yoga studios are founded by a person who has a need for the studio. These needs can be conscious and readily apparent, such as the need to grow and share a particular lineage or system of yoga. Or they could be subconscious and not readily apparent, such as the need to start a school in order to gather people together in a room in order to take their energy. This may sound like utter fantasy, but unfortunately, in my experience, it is not.

Let's take the example of a young child who seeks the love of his parents but whose parents give their love to him only when he behaves in a particular way, such as when he is playful or full of laughter, or when he comes back from kindergarten with a painting of mommy and daddy, or when he tells funny stories, puts on a show, sings a song, does a dance, or gives a performance. Although the child doesn't realize it, what he is doing is trading a particular type of energy in return for the energy of love from his parents. If the child has a deep need for love from his parents, he will need to trade a lot of his playful, creative, performing energy in return for this love. If the child's need for parental love is never properly fulfilled, the cycle of energy-trading becomes a fixed pattern of behavior in the child in his unending attempt to fulfill his need for parental love.

The energy needed to play, perform, sing a song, or create a painting of mommy and daddy comes from the second chakra, the chakra that governs creativity and artistic performance. But as the child grows into adulthood, this energy center evolves and develops to include energies that give rise to other forms of personal expression, such as sexuality. The child, now an adult, continues to need to trade their second-chakra energy in return for unfulfilled parental love. In adulthood, this becomes the trading of sexual energy in return for a form of parental love. If the need for love continues to be great, then the need for sexual energy continues to be great, as this is the energy needed for the trade.

If you are a yoga teacher and your own levels of personal sexual energy are low or are becoming depleted, you need to find an additonal source of sexual energy; you may need the sexual energy of other people. Mind you, this is all subconscious. If this is the case, you will take sexual energy from other people and use it to fulfill your own subconscious, unfulfilled early-childhood needs. This is a very simple cycle of trade based on need. However, in most adults it is a need originating in childhood that is long forgotten and has turned into a subconscious desire, and so the actions taken to fulfill this need have become subconscious too.

This is why it is not unusual to find a person setting up a yoga studio to fulfill a subconscious need for energy, and sometimes this energy is sexual energy. Their need is to be in a classroom full of people where a lot of sexual energy is generated and released into the classroom, for example in a kundalini, tantra, or biodanza class. The yoga studio owner, who is usually the principal teacher in the classroom, then draws this energy into his second chakra, giving it a boost in energy, which he then trades with his parents or parental figures for hoped-for love energy. I repeat: this is not a conscious process; it is totally subconscious.

If, as a student, you are happy to share or trade your sexual energy in return for yoga teachings, then you are in alignment with the energetic need of that particular studio. In return, the yoga teacher will reward you with his best attention. If you are not happy to share or trade your sexual energy in return for yoga, then you are out of alignment with the founding energy of the yoga studio and you might find that you do not quite fit in at that studio or class, or that the teacher doesn't give you as much attention as he gives others.

Attending a yoga studio that is designed to take your sexual energy ends up doing exactly that: as a student you may find that after a while you have less energy for sex, or that you feel less sexually confident in yourself. It is not the yoga that is causing you to feel this way; it is the subconscious needs of the yoga teacher.

Just be aware that some yoga studios have a subconscious energetic need of you, and that if you are not in alignment with that need, you will not fully integrate with that studio or teacher.

The same applies to aligning yourself with the energy of a massage therapist. Many massage therapists have a subconscious need, or reason, for doing what they do. These needs often merge with the subconscious needs of their clients. The needs are often harmless, like the need to learn about their own inner self through working with others, or the need to be told how good they are at what they do. But sometimes these needs are harmful, like the need for inappropriate touching, or the need to take some form of energy from you.

A yoga teacher may also have a subconscious need of their individual students, but in a classroom situation and without direct personal contact it is more difficult to discern what type of subconscious needs, if any, a teacher may have of you. Sometimes it takes years for a yoga teacher's subconscious needs from their students, such as sexual access, to reveal itself.

Thankfully, these scenarios are the exceptions in the wider yoga-teacher and massage-therapist community, where the vast majority of people do what they do out of love for what they do or out of respect for the lineage or system of yoga or bodywork they follow.

### Sensing Sick Sexual Energy

There is sometimes a problem in massage when either massage practice or massage training is used to gain inappropriate sexual access to another person, especially if the sexual access gained is without consent. I have seen it happen when teaching Thai massage in the Lahu village with Asokananda. In the middle of a large class of students there can be a single male (usually midlife or slightly older) who very subtly touches women inappropriately during massage practice.

The warning sign to look for in someone who uses sexual energy inappropriately is the person who makes you feel sick or yucky when they touch you, trying to connect with you in a way you are not expecting, in a way that makes you feel uncomfortable. This is someone whose sexual energy has been made sick by long-term inappropriate use, and you sense the sickness of their energy the moment they touch you. Sometimes they don't even have to touch you. People with severely sick sexual energy can also make you feel horrible even when you meet them in social situations.

If you ever feel this happening in a massage, you should stop the session immediately. Don't worry about offending the therapist; this is about protecting yourself, although be forewarned that therapists who are trying to get something extra from you will get very annoyed with you when you block the supply of what they subconsciously want from you.

## *Reading Your Teacher: The Four Energy Types*

Every teacher uses energy to teach; however, not every teacher uses the same energy in teaching. Knowing the different types of energy that teachers use can be important, as it can help guide you toward the teacher who is best suited to you and to what you want to achieve from your course of study. To read the energy of a teacher, you may have to spend some time with them in close quarters, for instance, at a weekend workshop or seminar, so that you can observe the teacher over the course of a few days.

When it comes to teachers, there are four basic energetic types:

### The Sexual-Energy Teacher

This is the teacher who brings the qualities of fun, play, pleasure, and the senses to the classroom and to their teaching. Fluid, flowing, yielding, moving, free, dancing, playful, experimental, humorous, musical, and even sensual, the teacher who brings any of these characteristics to the classroom is the teacher using second-chakra orange energy in their teaching. These can be classes of great excitement and anticipation and can make learning any system of yoga or massage an easy, wonderful, and pleasurable experience. This is an orange-energy teacher.

The only note about an orange teacher is that sometimes there can be a component of sexual energy in their teaching. Although what they teach is valuable and correct, a few orange teachers teach with the conscious intention of gaining sexual access to their students. In most cases this is not a problem, as the intention is conscious, so any sexual interplay that might result is usually well-signaled, and with the consent of both parties if undertaken. If, however, you feel uncomfortable in such a teaching environment, just make your sexual boundaries clear.

## The Intellectual-Energy Teacher

The intellectual-energy teacher makes for an ideal teacher as they tend to have a style that is clearly defined and very easy to follow. They stay on-point and never vary what they teach, making it very easy for the student to learn. They can sometimes, however, give you a headache in class from using too much intellectual energy in their teaching. The teaching is too rational, rigid, authoritarian, conformist, scientific, or methodological. The overall energy in the classroom is dry, with only limited warmth and moisture from shared personal experience, limited reference to spirituality, and not much playfulness. The imbalance of energy coming from an overabundance of intellectual energy, which is a yellow, air energy, is the cause of the headache.

A teacher who uses intellectual energy in the classroom may also reveal someone who is copying the knowledge of others without ever having directly experienced and understood what it is they are teaching. This might, for example, include the massage teacher who shows you therapy points and treatments that they have never used themselves. When you ask this teacher for the proof of what they teach, they will always refer to the book, to their own teacher, or to other teachers following the same system. They don't have the answers. No matter how much information the intellectual teacher gives you—and they will give you a lot—you sometimes intuitively feel that it is not enough, that there is something missing from their teaching. There is a part of you left wanting more. This is a very yellow experience. There is nothing wrong with what the intellectual-energy teacher is teaching; it's only that the energy with which they teach is a bit dry.

The teacher who gives you a headache could also be a warning sign that this person is trying to exert control over you. What the controlling teacher teaches may be valuable—it almost always is—but the energy with which they share this valuable information, their intention, is muddled. In its extreme form, the energy of control feels oppressive and can get strongly blocked in your head, neck, and shoulder tops. In a classroom, the energy of a teacher's need to exert control comes in through your ears and is mixed with the energy of wisdom in the words he or she uses. From there it descends down through your head, past your heart, and into your third chakra, the seat of intellectual understanding. It may be that your heart will have the deeper awareness that this energy is harmful to you and so blocks it in its downward descent through your body, causing a buildup and blockage of this energy in your head. This blockage causes headache. One of the ways to release the trapped energy of control from your head is to pull the energy back out through your ears. Imagine you have hair about six inches in length growing horizontally out of your ears. Grasp the hair with your hands and quickly pull it out. Repeat the exercise quickly twenty or thirty times. While doing the exercise you could imagine the face of the teacher who has given you the headache and tell him: "I know what you are doing. You're not going to get me like that." Alternatively you can seek out an appropriately trained shaman or energy worker to do this work for you.

A teacher who causes you a headache with their teaching can also reveal someone who is confused or conflicted, someone who does not fully understand what it is they are teaching. It may also reveal someone with a hidden degree of mental unhealthiness or imbalance.

On the plus side—and it is a big plus—intellectual-energy teachers, or schools that employ this type of teacher, are usually excellent at business, advertising, marketing, and promotion. The center where we store the energy necessary for intellectually based teaching, the third chakra, is also the center that houses the energy necessary for business and money. Teachers who use high levels of third-chakra energy in their teaching have the potential to run yoga or massage as a business and often do so very successfully. If your intention is to have yoga or massage as a successful business, seek out these third-chakra teachers and learn as much as possible from them.

## The Heart-Energy Teacher

The teacher who can you make you cry with empathy and understanding through stories from their own personal experience is sharing from the heart. You can feel the heart energy of such a teacher resonate in your own heart. It can make you catch your breath, instantly remind you of an episode in your own life, or bring tears to your eyes. If your teacher resonates in your heart like this, it is your heart telling you that what your teacher is teaching is true. It is a complete message, delivered with full understanding. There is nothing missing, unlike the feeling you sometimes get from a yellow intellectual-energy teacher. There is no need for rational, scientific proof of what the heart-centered teacher teaches. It *is* truth. This is the teacher of note.

Another aspect of the heart is that it is the seat of full understanding. This is why a teacher using heart energy is able to explain often complex issues in very simple terms. They can do so because they have a deep understanding of what they teach. The intention of a heart-energy teacher is to share the wisdom of experience and to use this wisdom to empower the student. They give freely, without expectations. Their teaching sets you free. It gives you strength. The heart-energy teacher also has the energy with which to create a strong feeling of family among the students in their classroom.

The down side, if you want to call it that, to the teacher who uses mostly heart energy in their yoga or massage teaching is that they tend to be poor at handling business and money. It is not their natural energy. They are often not very good at advertising themselves. This is why the heart-centered teacher can be difficult to find, as they get drowned out by the big and clever advertising of the business-oriented yellow yoga and massage teachers.

## The Spiritual-Energy Teacher

The spiritual-energy teacher is the person with the ability to bring people together who often do not know why they are going to this teacher in the first place. This is the energy of the underlying interconnectedness of life. As a student, you initially think you are going to study with this person to learn a certain something, but then later, when the class or workshop is over, you realize that the big thing you got from the class was that you met someone who then introduced you to a new book or person or situation that is now playing an influential part in your life. This is the energy of the spiritual teacher: the ability to bring the right people together, the ability to reveal the hidden interconnectedness among us.

The spiritual-energy teacher can also make you cry, but in a different way than the way the heart-energy teacher does. The heart-energy teacher makes you cry with a story of personal experience that resonates with something that relates to your own life. The spiritual-energy teacher can tell you a story that touches something much deeper inside you. It can cut through in a way you do not rationally understand, such as with a story you *feel* is true but yet you don't understand *why* it is true. When something touches this deeper level of inner understanding and truth, it is like touching your soul—it can make you cry. It is not the words of the story that cut through you; it is the energy used to carry those words to you, a high-level spiritual energy that has awakened a similar high-level energy within yourself. This is the energy of hidden inner wisdom, and when awakened, it can trigger experiences of deep insight and inspiration. The experience of inspiration may not be immediate. It takes a while for the energy of spiritual inspiration to travel through the body into the heart, where the energy passing through the heart triggers a *eureka!* moment. When this energy then enters your third chakra, it triggers the conscious understanding of what you need to do next in life. It is not unusual to attend the workshop of a spiritual-energy teacher and then "get it" six months later.

The down side of the spiritual-energy teacher is that their teachings sometimes stay in your head and you can lose them shortly afterward. Their classes often lack playfulness, dance, or movement. They lack orange energy. The energy of movement, dance, or play is essential in spiritual teaching, as physical movement is needed to move the high-level spiritual energy downward through the body, from where it first enters the body through the ears and the sixth chakra, to the lower centers of understanding, know-how, will, and action.

## The Energy of Cults

It is not uncommon to find a yoga teacher or yoga studio being a completely innocent ambassador for a yoga cult. Some systems of yoga are initially and very consciously born out of cult energy. To the novice students of the system, and indeed sometimes to the teachers of such a system, the cultish aspects are never visible or tangible. The only way to discern the presence of cult in the teachings of such a yoga teacher or studio is to dowse or otherwise read the energy of that teacher or studio. Cultish energy is very distinctive: dark steel gray in color, with a metaphysical feeling of heaviness and coldness.

Dark steel gray energy is the signature of cult and cannot be mistaken for anything else. I have given healing massages to innocent students of cult yoga and have found this heavy, tiring, sticky energy residing in various parts of their bodies. The energy can be in the second chakra if the student has had a sexual relationship with a teacher of the cult yoga. It can be in the root chakra if part of the teachings of the cult yoga involve exerting control over the student's sexual practice through strict mulabhanda (root chakra) exercises. It can also be in the head or in the third chakra if the teacher mixes the energy of the cult with the energy of wisdom in the words he or she is using in their teachings.

Again—and it must be repeated here—some teachers are completely unaware that the system of yoga they follow and teach is born out of cult energy, and that they are innocently passing this energy on to their students through their teachings. I would also like to stress that most forms of sexual-energy discipline in yoga, such as mulabhanda exercises, are there for the purpose of positive advancement in yoga practice and are not harmful to the student in any way. If, as a yoga student, you feel unsure of the intention of your teacher in their teaching certain aspects of yoga involving sexual energy, use the services of a shaman, energy worker, or spiritual healer and have them read the energies of your chakras. If your chakra energies are in a healthy state, if they correspond to the clear colors of the rainbow, then so is your yoga practice, and so too are the teachings of your teacher.

That which gives a cult its strength and holds it together is its energy. And the energy of cult is a spider's web. A cult is started by one person with the intention of trapping other people into it. It links an entire community, and if you get caught in it, it can be very difficult to break free of. Cult energy is spread between people in various ways: through pseudospiritual or intellectual teachings, by engaging in shared rituals, through direct authority and control, or through sexual contact. Regardless of the reason and purpose of a cult or the methodology used in spreading it, the energy used to maintain it is always the same: dark steel gray in color, and heavy, sticky, and tiring in feeling.

The same applies to lodges or secret brotherhoods. They use a specific energy to build and hold together their community. The ways this energy is spread among its members are the same ways cult energy is spread through a yoga cult. The only difference is in the type of energy that is used. One well-known lodge, which has nothing to do with yoga, uses a very specific energy to bind its members together. It is a dark indigo energy that has the presence of black smoke mixed with it. It also uses a particular energy as a "fixing agent," to subvert and contain this energy so it can be spread among a closed circle of people. The fixing-agent energy is a mixture of silver and crystal white energy and is of a very high vibration. In this respect, there is no difference between a spell, hex, or curse that uses a crow's foot as a fixing agent and the energy used among the members of a lodge or secret brotherhood that uses white crystal energy as a fixing agent. Dark indigo energy is a high form of indigo energy, the energy of the sixth chakra. It is a light but very powerful energy form, and when released into the body it gives rise to temporary feelings of great confidence, power, and ability. It is a predominantly male energy, and because of its color it reveals itself as an energy not of this Earth, but one that has traveled to Earth from a distant, faraway place. Because it is an energy that can travel great distances, dark indigo energy is in and of itself an expansive energy that carries great freedom with it. It is free to come and go. It is free to stay or leave. It is free to travel wherever it wishes. However, this aspect of the energy, its freedom, is of no use to the brotherhood that seeks to harvest and control it for the purpose of using it for personal gain among a closed community. The indigo energy is therefore purposely tempered and controlled by the silver and crystal white energy. This causes hurt and pain to the indigo energy, and it is this hurt and pain within the indigo that is revealed by the presence of black smoke.

Lodge energy is neither metaphysically heavy nor light, hot nor cold. When released, it causes the body to feel a slight tension and tightness.

By complete contrast, it does not give rise to feelings of expansion and freedom, which true dark indigo energy gives rise to. Its energy does give rise to some feelings of confidence, power, and ability, but due to the use of the fixing agent, the silver and crystal white energy, only a tiny fraction of the energy's true potential is experienced.

Although lodge or secret brotherhood energy can indeed be used in the creation of personal gain, there are three aspects to it that are inseparable in its use:

1. You will lose your freedom. The energy that you use for your personal gain is not free. It has been tempered and controlled. By integrating something into yourself that has been tempered and controlled, you too will be tempered and controlled. You may as well give up on any notion you have of becoming a free person, as you have already, unknowingly, lost this freedom.

2. You will be controlled. The energy of a lodge that is used for personal gain should be, by its nature, free to come and go. In its natural state it travels and passes through everything. Its effects are naturally fleeting and temporary. The energy that you use for personal gain, however, is not free. It has had its freedom taken away from it, and it is bound and held in slavery. When you integrate such an energy into your own body, you too become bound and held in slavery. You are, from that moment on, controlled.

3. You will experience pain. The lodge energy that you use for your personal gain is suffering because part of it has been sabotaged, bound, and enslaved. By integrating something into your body that is in pain, you too will experience some degree of metaphysical or physical pain in your body.

### How People Are Lured into Lodges and Cults

Some people are singled out by lodges and cults to serve as recruiting officers to seek out new members. Some of these people are aware of their role as recruiting officers, and so there is no problem. Sometimes, however, these people may be unaware that they are being used as recruiting officers. Indeed, some recruiting officers are not even members of the particular cult they are being used as a recruiting officers for. Oftentimes these recruiting officers are women with strong sexual energy. Somewhere in their history they have had sexual contact with a member of the cult, and through this intimacy the energy of the cult was passed into the body of the woman. This energy, now residing in the woman, then seeks out other people, mostly male, who will potentially match the needs of the energy of the cult or brotherhood. The problem is that many of these female recruiting officers are completely unaware that they are carrying the energy of the lodge/cult within their body, and that they are being used as recruiting officers.

What happens is that the woman becomes unconsciously drawn to potential new members, and potential new members find themselves unconsciously drawn to her. This sometimes leads to confusion. She may find that she is attracting men to her that fit the needs of the lodge or cult, yet she herself is not attracted to these men. Or she might find a man to whom she is attracted, but that man's energy may not fit the needs of the cult. When she does unconsciously attract a potential new member whom she is also attracted to, and where there is a close enough fit between the needs of the cult and the needs of the potential new member, then the energy of the cult gets passed from the recruiting officer to the potential new member, usually through intimate contact, so that the cult or lodge expands its membership. The newly recruited member may subsequently find himself unconsciously drawn to the group, while at the same time members of the group may find themselves unconsciously drawn to the potential new recruit.

As with any community held together with energy such as that of a lodge or cult, the connection to the community can be undone by an appropriate energy worker, shaman, or spiritual healer able to identify the type of energy being used to hold the group together.

## Taking on Bad Energy in Massage

Opinion is greatly divided on the subject of whether we can take on the bad energy of a massage client, or simply take on bad energy from people in general. Some people believe you can, others say you cannot. When I first started my career in massage I was one of the believers, but I now know, in heart and spirit, that I do not take on bad energy from clients in massage.

When I first started out in Thai massage, I had no experience or understanding of energy whatsoever. It was mentioned briefly in class, but the concept of energy was never properly discussed or explored. I did my massage believing that that was all it was: massage, the physical manipulation of the body of another person. Everything went well for the first few months until at the end of one massage I felt a lot more tired than usual. That was the start. I soon found that I was getting tired more frequently. The cumulative effect of such tiredness began to leave me more and more vulnerable to tiredness. Sensing the vulnerability, I began to practice protection exercises. I noticed I felt more tired after difficult massages, or massages with clients who were carrying difficult issues. Feeling well before such a massage and then feeling tired, exhausted, or sometimes nauseous after the massage led me to conclude that I was somehow taking on bad energy from clients. Not knowing if this was the case or not, I checked in with some of my contemporaries to find out whether they were experiencing similar feelings. The generally accepted theory was we were all taking on bad energy from our clients. This is what was making us tired. With nothing else to counter this generalization, I accepted it as my personal belief too.

The undoing of this belief was so gradual and subtle that I was not aware it was happening at the time. I was four years into my massage career when I experienced a very deep spiritual connection with a client and suddenly saw the other side of the debate. It was also the moment I was able to look back on the previous four years and recognize some anomalies in the pattern of taking on bad energy. These anomalies were clues that pointed to the truth: that you do not take on the bad energy of your client. I wish to share these anomalies with you now, in the hope they may persuade you to revisit your own belief that you can take on the bad energy of a massage client.

One thing I noticed was how some of my clients were remarkably easier for me to treat than others. At the time I was curious enough to ask about the lives of those easy clients to find out why they even needed massage. One massage in particular was so easy for me, it was as effortless as slicing a hot knife through butter. Due to my ongoing training in energy work at the time, I had an inkling that this particular client's body pain had something to do with his brother. And indeed it did. He had held in his body years of jealousy of his older brother who, when he left school, was allowed to go on to study at a university, while my client, the younger brother, was denied this opportunity and forced to take a job to support the family. This was a major lightbulb moment in my massage work. I am a single child. I have no brothers and no sisters, therefore I could not relate to the pain of jealousy of an older sibling. The pain was alien to me, and when in my massage I released the energy of this pain from the body of my client, it found nothing within my own body or energy system to resonate with or hook on to. The energy of my client's pain, when released, simply dissolved into the atmosphere of my massage studio. I could not take it on because there was nothing within me by which it could be taken in.

Another time I was to receive a new male client. I arrived early at my workplace and got everything ready. I sat quietly to relax and do a little prayer and meditation. After a few minutes, I suddenly began to feel queasy. This was an unexpected and unwanted first. The feeling did not subside; it intensified. By the time my client arrived, I was ashen, sweaty, and dehydrated. I had no idea what was happening. I gathered myself together and started the massage. It was awful. I had to stop at regular intervals to gather my strength and center. The entire treatment was a nightmarish struggle. When I finished, I offered my apologies to my client, saying I was not in my best form. He said he felt it in me. We began to talk.

It transpired that he had been badly treated by his mother when he was very young, and that after years of holding the energies of maltreatment by his mother in his body, he was now seeking release from his past, and was coming to me as part of his rehabilitation. His story struck me like a ton of bricks. I too had been maltreated by my mother, and at that point in my massage career I was only beginning to realize the depth of adverse effects it had had on my life and on my body. This is why this particular massage was so difficult for me and why it caused me to feel sick, exhausted, and heavy. My client was carrying the same hurt in his body as I was carrying in mine. When I accessed the energy of his pain through the action of massage, I was at the same time accessing the energies of my own forgotten, unreleased pain. At that point I intuitively understood that massages I found to be the most difficult and draining were massages in which the clients were carrying the same issues I had in my own life, issues I had either buried or forgotten, and most definitely had not dealt with or released.

Two or three summers following this most difficult massage experience, I was in the middle of a very enjoyable treatment with a client who was a longstanding yoga practitioner. The person's body was soft, warm, and yielding and was making the massage a complete delight. I felt completely set free by my client and took the opportunity to let go, both in my mind and in my body. Without any expectation, and working with eyes closed, fully immersed in the moment, I suddenly found myself in a space where I felt there were no physical boundaries between my client and me. It felt like I was no longer bound by the form of a physical body. At the same time I found that I was unable to recognize a physical form for the body of my massage client. Neither of us were bodies. Without the physical form of body, there was also no boundaries or separation between us. I had somehow transcended the three-dimensional reality of two separated beings placed within a fixed location. With no reference of physical form to rely on, I experienced that my massage client and I were formless energies in an unending universe of moving, plasmalike energy. We were no longer bodies, we were energy, slightly denser forms of energy within an endless soup of energy. It felt as if I were an extension of my client and that my client were an extension of me. It was a moment of astonishing spiritual insight. In that moment of feeling one with my massage client, I realized that if I am one with my massage client, then I cannot take on the bad energy of a client, as there is no "other" to take bad energy on from!

As long as your experience in massage is that of duality, you will believe in the phenomenon of taking on bad energy. When your experience transcends duality, that belief is shattered.

## Spells, Hexes, and Curses

Just as excitement is a form of sexual energy, anger a form of emotional energy, ambition a form of mental energy, intuition a form of spiritual energy, and extreme control a form of cult energy, so are spells, hexes, and curses forms of energy.

Spells, hexes, and curses are forms of energy that can be used to create blockages in any part of a person's energy system, and they can be difficult to break. The scope of a spell and its effect is extremely wide. It can range from someone thinking ill of you, to someone giving you the evil eye, to someone praying that misfortune happens you (as exemplified in "Hidden Forms of Hurt to Women's Sexual Energy," pages 145–49). In other examples, people employ the services of a shaman, witch doctor, or spiritualist to create a spell. A spell is a form of energy that can be sent to or cast on someone, causing them to experience some form of blockage, disease, or illness, such as casting a green octopus energy spell on a person's chest, resulting in that person suffering a bout of bronchitis.

Although I am not skilled in the use of magic, I have great respect for that type of energy. It may seem completely fanciful to some of you, but it is not. There is, however, a link between your belief in the use of magic and the effects that magic can have on you. For instance, if you are a tourist in a city where there is a strong use of magic by local shamans, there may be parts of that city where local people will not walk at night due to the adverse effects of the general, prevailing magic. But a tourist with no awareness of such magic can walk through that area without experiencing any adverse side effects. If you have no awareness of the energy of local magic, then that energy has nothing to hold on to in you. It can also be said that the magic is not meant to influence you as you are not the target audience.

People who use spells, hexes, and curses are people who have been trained to connect with and use these particular types of energy. It is no more mysterious than the successful businessman who has been trained to connect with and use the energy of his third chakra, the energy that is necessary for business and the creation of wealth. Some people create magic, some people create business success. Both are creations of energy.

Spells, hexes, and curses are said to be powerful forms of energy, but as forms of energy they are no more or no less powerful than the sexual energy that enables a person to have sex or the mental, willpower energy that helps a student concentrate on a course of study. Spells, hexes, and curses are said to be powerful because their knowledge is held by a small group of people who, by controlling access to and use of these energies, remain in a position of perceived power. In some of the world's indigenous populations where the use of magic is part of everyday life, the use of spells, hexes, and curses is no more mysterious than apples growing on an apple tree.

Spells, hexes, and curses are normally judged to be cast by non-holy people, but some spells, such as ecclesiastical spells, have been cast throughout history by agents of a church or religious organization.

Whereas some forms of energy—sexual energy, mental willpower energy, and the energy of love—are to be found within the physical body, much of the energy used in spells, hexes, and curses belong outside the realm of the physical body and requires specific training to find and use effectively. Such energies can be described as belonging to otherworldly entities, star systems, or dimensions. The energy is channeled by trained channelers from otherworldly dimensions into our everyday three-dimensional world, where it is used to varying effect. Some of these energies are put into symbolic shells so they can be more easily manipulated. Three symbolic shells that I have come across are the chicken's foot, the octopus, and a black, eyeless, fishlike creature. They are metaphysical shells that hold the energy of magic within, just as our body is the physical shell that houses our biological energies within.

The adverse physical, emotional, mental, or spiritual effects of a spell, hex, or curse can always be undone. This is accomplished by setting free the energy that is housed in the symbolic shell or form and sending it back home, to its appropriate origin. This process requires the services of a trained shaman, energy worker, spiritual healer, or exorcist. In some methods, angels and archangels are used to dispel the hex energies.

You may ask how this is relevant to a person following a path of yoga, but if you are on a path of yoga that has brought you to a strongly spiritual place or community, it may happen that you have become hexed because you have somehow shown an inappropriate attitude, lack of proper understanding, or lack of respect to the spirits or energies present where you have been studying. For instance, in some spiritual communities where you go to learn meditation, yoga, or massage, it may be appropriate to make an offering to the spirits of the teachers and students who have preceded you, the sangha. If you do not do this, the spirits present may give you a "clip across the back of the head" in the form of a small hex, for not showing proper respect. The hex or spell can then be used to block either your mind or your body from opening deeper into your practice. This is why in some forms of remedying a hex or spell, the person who has been hexed has to bring an offering to a particular place of worship or to a particular spirit. The offering is to the spirit or energy originally disrespected. Such an offering of recognition is often enough to appease the spirit, which then releases its energy from the symbolic form of the spell cast on the person. Always remember to be respectful of the spirits, energies, and spiritual traditions encountered along your path.

Energy is just energy. It can be of different frequency or vibration. Energies of differing vibrations have differing effects on the biological organism of the human body. Energy that vibrates at one specific frequency that is labeled "sexual" causes feelings of arousal and excitement. Energy of another frequency, labeled "anger," causes the body to harden, tighten, and clench. Another frequency, labeled "inspiration," causes the brain to form ideas. One energy frequency is called "Angel Gabriel" and causes feelings of peace and spiritual happiness. Yet another, different frequency is called "cult" and links people together. Take away the words, the labels, the explanations, and all you are left with is energy,

energy that has different effects on the mind and body depending on its frequency, or vibration. If you discount one form of energy and the effect it has on the mind and body simply because you cannot see it, feel it, experience it, or rationally explain it, then you have to discount all other forms of energy. If you discount the healing effects of spiritual energy, then you have to discount the arousing effects of sexual energy, for both are, in essence, the same thing, energy, the only difference being that one is vibrating at a slightly different frequency than the other. It is the same as green and red. You cannot discount one color and accept another. You either accept both, or discount both. They're both the same thing—they're both forms of light. They're both forms of energy.

---

### Prana Egg for Protection

If you are working on someone in massage whose energy field disturbs you in some way, you have two options: center and ground yourself after the massage or, perhaps better yet, create some form of protection for yourself before the massage, such as a prana egg. You create a prana egg by visualizing the highest color, purple, and using it to build an egglike form of protection around yourself. This gives temporary protection against all energy levels below purple, which account for about 98 percent of most people you will ever see in massage. Don't forget to fill yourself, your own body, with the color purple too. For even more complete protection, gold is said to be the best energy color to use when filling your prana egg. Note that the effect of another person's energy field touching or passing through yours is temporary and not permanent. Feeling the energetic presence of the Dalai Lama does not turn you into the Dalai Lama.

---

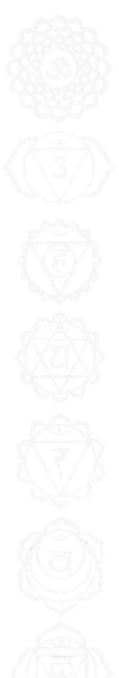

# PART THREE

# Healing Emotional Blockages

# 7

# Reading the Colors of Energy

This is a practical guide for those studying their own energy and for yoga practitioners, massage therapists, and energy healers who are beginning to become sensitive to the colors of energy in their practice or their lives and seek help in interpreting the meaning of the colors they are sensing or seeing. This is not a comprehensive guide to all the meanings of all the possibilities for colors of energy, a subject that is beyond the scope of this book. Rather, it is intended as an overview and introduction to the colors of commonly found energies, along with typical energy blockages associated with those colors, which can be seen, felt, or intuited especially during a massage treatment or yoga practice.

We know that energies in different parts of the body, specifically the main energy centers, or chakras, vibrate at different frequencies. For example, the energy of the first chakra vibrates at a frequency that is red in color. The first chakra also houses energies of different colors, reflective of the seven different layers within the chakra. When the first chakra is in a healthy state, the colors of the seven layers can be seen as the seven colors of a rainbow, so when a color in a chakra is described as rainbow red, it means the shade of red as seen in a rainbow. However, nonrainbow colors, such as black, gray, or brown, can sometimes be seen in a chakra, revealing the presence of an energy that is causing blockage in the chakra. Similarly an overly strong presence of a particular rainbow color in a chakra can reveal a state of imbalance caused by an excess of one particular energy, or color. For example, a significant presence of yellow within the normally green color of the heart chakra reveals an overly strong presence of yellow energy, which is associated with third-chakra mental energy. This indicates a person who lives more in the world of intellect and less in the world of love, and this preference of intellect over matters of the heart is causing hurt to the heart, which may manifest in a condition of physical tightness or tension in the chest area housing the heart.

A basic understanding of the meanings of the colors can help you first and foremost in forming a diagnosis or evaluation of the underlying energetic cause of any condition of physical discomfort or unease in your own body, and then in the body of a massage client or yoga student. A skilled color-reader is able to discern the health and balance of energy throughout a person's entire body and is easily able to sense where pain or blockage resides in certain chakras, simply by ascertaining its color.

I have given more attention to the non-rainbow colors of energy in this chapter. As a healer, massage therapist, or energy worker, you will tend to encounter more people who are unwell than those who are well. It is therefore helpful to be familiar with the colors of unease, disease, blockage, and pain, whether in oneself or someone you are working on.

## OVERVIEW OF COLORS

| PRINCIPAL COLOR | VARIATIONS AND COMBINATIONS |
|---|---|
| Red | None |
| Orange | Orange and **Gray** |
| | Orange and **Lavender** |
| Yellow | None |

## OVERVIEW OF COLORS (continued)

| PRINCIPAL COLOR | VARIATIONS AND COMBINATIONS |
|---|---|
| Green | Bright Yellow Green |
| | Dark Green |
| | Yellow and Green |
| Blue | Sky Blue |
| | Royal Blue |
| | Indigo |
| Purple | Red and Purple |
| | Green and Purple |
| | Deep Purple |
| | Violet and Ultraviolet |
| | Lavender |
| Black | Red and Black |
| | Orange and Black |
| | Yellow and Black |
| | Green and Black |
| | Sky Blue and Black |
| | Gray and Black |
| | Indigo and Black |
| White | Sky Blue and White |
| Gray | Light or Pale Gray |
| | Steel Gray |
| | Deep Gray or Dark Gray |
| | Dark Steel Gray |
| Brown | Golden Brown or Honey Brown |
| | Dark Brown |

## Red

Red is a positive, healthy color. When you sense the color red in your own body or in the body of a massage client or yoga student, it usually indicates any of the following:

Strength
Groundedness
Family
Goddess energy
The energy of female love
The physical body
The first chakra

Wearing red clothes generates feelings of strength and confidence. Red is also a good color to wear when someone needs grounding, especially red socks or red shoes.

## Orange

When you sense the color orange in your own body or in the body of another person, it usually indicates the energy of the second chakra or sexual energy. Healthy sexual energy is rainbow orange in color. When sexual energy has been damaged or hurt, the orange will be mixed with another color, usually gray or black (see the relevant sections in this chapter). Sometimes the gray or black and orange appear as two colors clearly seen side-by-side, while other times it appears as if gray or black has been mixed with the orange, resulting in an overall dirty orange or dark orange color.

Wearing orange generates sexual energy. However, because human sexual energy has, in general, become damaged and hurt through thousands of years of abuse and misuse, orange can be a difficult or uncomfortable color for most people to wear. Usually, only people with clean and healthy sexual energy can comfortably wear orange.

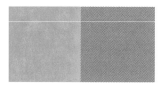

### Orange and Gray

The two colors orange and gray, when seen side-by-side, reveal someone who is insecure with their sexual energy, is unclear about sexual energy, or doesn't fully trust sexual energy.

### Orange and Lavender

Orange and lavender seen side-by-side indicate someone who needs to have greater awareness of their sexual energy. This may be because they do not understand the patterns of behavior carried in sexual energy. An example of this is the person who gives their sexual energy to another, usually in the act of sex, in the hope of receiving love in return; this lack of awareness has led the person to being constantly manipulated and hurt by others in adult sexual relationships. The presence of lavender in this instance reveals the person's need for lavender energy, and by using lavender in your healing work, you will help bring the energy of greater awareness to this person's understanding of their sexual energy.

## Yellow

Yellow is a Jekyll and Hyde color. On the one hand it is the color of strong intellect, will, determination, ego, confidence, and ability. Its presence can reveal enormous warmth, happiness, and radiance within a person. It is also a very powerful healing color. On the other hand, yellow is the most prevalent color of most energy blockages.

Yellow is the color associated with the energy of the third chakra and with the TCM meridians associated with the third chakra: the spleen, stomach, liver, and gallbladder meridians. From the third chakra springs the energy that carries our thoughts, beliefs, and patterns of behavior throughout our body, and it is those thoughts, beliefs, and patterns of behavior that create the widest range of energy blockages that result in hurt in the body.

The scope of yellow energy blockage is as vast as the scope of human thought—anything from the belief that you are a powerful person, capable of any achievement, and therefore have the right to mistreat anyone who gets in your way or who you believe is inferior to you, to the belief that you are a worthless, insecure being incapable of achieving even the smallest of feats.

Of the hundreds of different yellow-colored intellectual-energy blockages that can be found in the body, here are four common examples:

- **A yellow energy blockage originating in third chakra and found in the spleen meridian:** This indicates a blockage caused by the person their using their life-force energy in a way that is not aligned to its best use, for example, a person staying in a relationship in which there are no children and the relationship is well and truly over. The person's life-force energy is being wasted in a dead-end relationship, and this is causing a blockage in the flow of this energy in their spleen meridian. This then manifests as physical tension and tightness in the third chakra and in the areas of the body running close to the running of the spleen meridian.

- **A yellow energy blockage originating in the third chakra and found in the stomach meridian:** This may reveal a client's inability to ingest and digest forms of energy, including nutritional and environmental energy. Someone with a blockage in yellow stomach energy may be experiencing the harmful effects of an overbearing, bullying, or controlling person in their life. As an act of self-defense against such an overbearing influence, the person blocks off the energy of the overbearing or controlling person. This act of self-defense is then mirrored in a blockage in the ability to ingest other forms of energy, including nutritional energy from food. The person develops dietary sensitivities as a result. This form of self-defense gives rise to a blockage in the free flow of energy in the areas of the third chakra and the stomach, as well as in the areas of the body running close to the stomach meridian.

The blockage gives rise to the physical experience of tension and tightness in the stomach and upper abdominal area.

- **A yellow energy blockage originating in the third chakra and found in the liver meridian:** This reveals an excessive buildup of an emotional nature, such as anger, rage, frustration, or impatience. These emotional buildups can also found in the gallbladder meridian. A buildup of anger causes a energetic pressure along the liver meridian and can often manifest as an itch or irritable feeling on the inside of the thigh, a tightening in the groin, or an acidic pain behind the lower ribs. From personal experience, I have also found a correlation between childhood hernia operations and unexpressed childhood anger.

- **A yellow energy blockage originating in the third chakra and running along the gallbladder meridian:** This represents the greatest range of energy blockage, discomfort, pain, and disease stemming from the same, single issue: the person's beliefs about him- or herself. Blockages and physical pain relating to self-beliefs can be pervasive along the entire running of the gallbladder meridian, depending on the number and severity of self-held beliefs that the person has that run contrary to what is actually true. A strongly held belief such as "If I lose my job, my whole life will fall apart" is not only strong enough to paralyze a person's lifestyle, the energy it takes to hold on to this belief so strongly causes a parallel degree of physical paralysis or tightness in the body. The body areas most commonly affected by the energy of negative self-beliefs include the shoulders, the trapezius, the sides of the neck, below the armpits, along the outside of the rib cage, the solar plexus, across the outside of the gluteus maximus, and along the outsides of the thighs—in general, all the body areas close to the running of the gallbladder meridian.

Yellow is a powerfully energetic color to wear. It radiates self-belief and self-confidence but requires a certain amount of confidence and belief to be worn. Putting on yellow clothes can give you a shiver or thrill of energy. For some people, however, yellow can be a very unsettling color to wear, causing feelings of internal unease or discomfort.

## Green

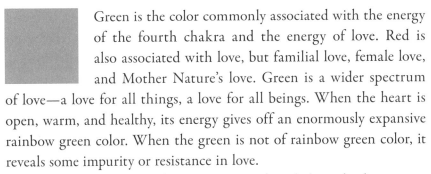

Green is the color commonly associated with the energy of the fourth chakra and the energy of love. Red is also associated with love, but familial love, female love, and Mother Nature's love. Green is a wider spectrum of love—a love for all things, a love for all beings. When the heart is open, warm, and healthy, its energy gives off an enormously expansive rainbow green color. When the green is not of rainbow green color, it reveals some impurity or resistance in love.

Green is a softening color to wear. It is also a balanced color to wear in as much as it neither radiates energy, like yellow, nor draws in energy, like black. It also brings a sense of calm.

### Bright Yellow Green

Bright yellow green, as in a green that is tinged with bright yellow, reveals the presence of the energy of jealousy: your jealousy of another person or another person's jealousy of you.

### Dark Green

Dark green indicates the presence of the energy of lovelessness, sorrow, or despair.

### Yellow and Green

The color combination of green and yellow side-by-side reveals the presence of love that is given on condition. In this example of a two-color energy blockage, yellow means control—in this case, love that is controlled.

## Sky Blue

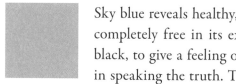

Sky blue reveals healthy, clear, truthful communication, completely free in its expression. Sky blue mixed with black, to give a feeling of dirty sky blue, indicates a fear in speaking the truth. The combination of sky blue and black side-by-side reveals someone searching for or needing the truth but who has yet to find it. They may be being blocked by someone else in their attempt to find it.

Sky blue is a very liberating color to wear. It gives a feeling of lightness, freedom, and space. Like green, wearing sky blue also creates a sense of calm and peace. I have found that people who like wearing sky blue, usually as a scarf, also like wearing lavender, another liberating, peaceful color.

### *Blue*
Blue is the color of everyday communication, not yet free enough to carry difficult truths, but strong enough for everyday use.

### *Royal Blue*
Royal blue is the color of a communication that is hidden, i.e., a secret. Royal blue can reveal someone who keeps a secret, and the pressure of keeping that secret is what is causing the person's distress. Alternatively, it can mean that there is something about the person's life that is being kept secret from her, and her not knowing the secret is causing a blockage and pain in her body. In healing work, be aware that you are not always allowed to release the energy of a secret, as the truth behind it may be too damaging to the person. If you are not allowed to release the secret, you will be unable to energetically connect with the royal blue energy.

## Indigo

Indigo is a high-vibration energy that brings spiritual understanding and healing. It is usually found in the area of the sixth chakra.

Sometimes you find indigo mixed with black, or indigo and black side-by-side as a two-color combination. This reveals either a fear of spiritual matters or that the person is at the limit of their spiritual understanding. This can be important to discern as it reveals that for the person to further deepen into their yoga practice they must focus more deeply on the spiritual aspects of practice. A lack of spiritual understanding of yoga practice can often lead to a blockage in the deepening of practice.

Wearing indigo clothes has the very subtle effect of making you feel you are not fully integrated with your surroundings. Indigo draws your focus away from yourself, moving your energy away from the conscious. Going grocery shopping while wearing indigo may make you forget one or two of the grocery items you went shopping for.

## Purple

Purple indicates the presence of a strong spiritual connection and a deep understanding of spiritual matters. Although it is usually associated with the seventh chakra, it can be found anywhere throughout the body. It is a powerful healing energy and can be used in any kind of energy healing or spiritual healing, in any part of the body. You can use it on yourself by meditating on the color purple and then metaphysically moving it around your body to where your body needs healing. Close your eyes. Bring an awareness of the color purple to your mind's eye and focus on it. When the purple is established, gently move your focus to a part of your body that needs healing. The purple will follow your focus to that body part. Keep the purple in the area that needs healing until its color dissipates. Repeat the exercise if you wish.

When working on another person, you can first meditate on the color purple to alter the balance of energy within your own system before you perform a healing on that person. You will then be able to transmit the purple energy to any part of your cleint's body through your touch.

Purple is a surprisingly powerful color to wear. Like red, it also gives feelings of strength and confidence, but the feelings are much more subtle.

### Red and Purple

Red with purple side-by-side is a very powerful color combination, the energies of heaven and earth brought together. When you see them in the body, it reveals activated first and seventh chakras, normally associated with people who have been working strongly on their self-healing or spiritual self-development.

Wearing the color combination of red and purple is the most energetically powerful combination I know, as you are symbolically bringing the energy of earth, red, together with the energy of heaven, purple. It is also fun to play with the order of the colors. There is a difference between wearing a purple top with red bottoms and wearing a red top with purple bottoms. In the latter combination, you are symbolically turning your life upside down!

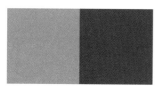

### Green and Purple

The combination of green with purple indicates a person whose source of love lies within the divine, as opposed to emotional love or familial love.

### Deep Purple

Deep purple indicates the presence of energy that has traveled to Earth from deep space. It sounds fanciful, but Earth, as a planet, is constantly being bombarded by energies traveling throughout the universe; sometimes these energies reach the surface of our planet and touch the energy system of a person. If you have deep purple in your energy system, you can sometimes dream about people you know, but in your dream they take on a slightly alien appearance, such as having blue skin or extra-large, dark eyes. These are just symbols our conscious mind uses in trying to categorize this particular type of energy when it is present in our energy system. Completely irrational and harmless, but great fun!

### Violet and Ultraviolet

The colors violet or ultraviolet reveal the presence of extremely powerful healing energy. Red, orange, yellow, and green are warming, strengthening, and healing colors, but as energies of a lower frequency and vibration they are slow-working in their effectiveness. Violet, and in particular ultraviolet, are of such a high frequency that they work much more quickly, almost violently so, in their healing effects. It is their higher frequency that enables these colors to break through energy blockages found in the first, second, and third chakras so effectively. Some spiritual healers working with the energies of the Ascended Masters use the energy of the violet flame of St. Germain in the healing of their clients.

Caution needs to be observed when working with ultraviolet energy, however. It is strong enough to cause your own energy system to partially short-circuit when you first connect to it or when you first use it as a healing color in your massage work. Meditating on the color ultraviolet can similarly cause powerful electricity-like feelings to rush through your energy meridians. If you are able to integrate ultraviolet energy into your massage work, it will bring enormous healing to your clients. It should be noted that some medical devices utilize the power of ultraviolet light to help repair damaged body tissue.

### Lavender

Lavender is the color of energy that brings answers to the confusions of life. It is used as a healing energy when working with a person who is confused or lost and lacks sufficient understanding as to why things have gone wrong or worked out the way they have. If you see the color combination of yellow and lavender side-by-side in the body of a client you are working with, it reveals that the person you are working with needs lavender energy to be introduced into their crown and sixth chakras, and from there moved downward through their body to their third chakra. In this example the presence of lavender is indicative of the need for lavender. Lavender energy, being of a higher vibration than yellow, a conscious-mind energy, will raise the level of consciousness of the person, which in turn brings a greater understanding of life to the person. Lavender energy lessens feelings of confusion, while at the same time it opens the door to a higher understanding of life. Seeing the color lavender by itself, whether in your own mind's eye or in the body of another person, simply reveals the presence of lavender energy.

Although lavender is powerful enough to raise a person's level of intellect, it is a very soft and gentle color to use and has no adverse effects whatsoever. Paradoxically, it is an energy highly intellectual people are suspicious or afraid of.

## Black

 Black is the most difficult of all colors to interpret. It has a wide range of meanings, each of which is determined by the quality or texture of the blackness of the energy. Some of the textural variations are very subtle, so it takes many years of working with black to understand the differences. For example, black is the color of the energy of fear. Black is also the color of yin, female energy, which can be used in the healing of fear. So when you sense the presence of black energy in the body, consider which energy are you about to connect with: the energy of fear or the yin energy? Below are the most common meanings of black energy. I have added personal experiential descriptions of the quality and texture of each of the black energies, but these are for loose guidance only.

Yin, female energy (cool, black energy)

Spiritual, female, sexual-healing energy (cool, soft-feeling, fuzzy black energy of great depth)

Fear (usually cold to very cold in temperature, often sticky in feel, sometimes heavy like black motor oil, sometimes light, like black smoke)

Loneliness (cold, strongly opaque, obsidian or black ice-like in appearance)

Pain (cold, wet, slightly swollen, soft black energy)

Emptiness (black, as in the blackness in a huge, empty underground cavern)

The source of all thoughts and ideas (the blackness that lies beyond the edge of the universe)

The energy of not knowing, as in the words "I don't know what to do" (when you connect with this black, you get a strong and immediate sense of being personally mentally blocked)

Blockage (an author suffering writer's block will have a cloud of black smoky energy in their head, in their sixth chakra)

### Red and Black

If you sense the color combination red and black side-by-side in the body of a person, it can suggest one of the following:

- There is an area of black energy—pain—present within the red energy area of the person's body.
- The healthy advancement in the life of the person is being blocked by an issue in their red energy, their root chakra.
- The person is afraid of something red. This can be the red of their root chakra and may indicate something that happened in the person's earliest childhood. In some cases it reveals that the person is afraid of a member of their family, or even afraid of life.

The same methods of interpretation can be used when determining the meanings of the color combinations of orange and black, yellow and black, green and black, sky blue and black, and indigo and black seen side-by-side. The following are a few additional examples of two-color side-by-side combinations that include black. There are many more possible interpretations of such color combinations, so this is just an overview.

### Orange and Black

When orange appears with black, it indicates sexual energy that has been hurt. This is often found in the subtle-energy body of a woman who has suffered a miscarriage or abortion.

### Yellow and Black

Yellow and black side-by-side can indicate someone who has difficulty in dealing with money, such as a fear of money, as money is a very powerful form of yellow energy.

### Green and Black

Dirty green, as in green that is mixed with black in a single color, or alternatively, green and black seen side-by-side, reveals a blockage in the flow of love energy, a fear of love, or someone whose heart has been hurt. Maybe the person is afraid to love because they have been hurt in love before. The blockage in the flow of love energy can be in the receiving of love as well as in the giving of love. Dark, dirty green energy is most commonly found in the fourth chakra.

### Sky Blue and Black

Sky blue with black shows a person who is afraid to speak their truth, or a person from whom the truth is being hidden.

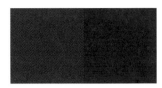

### Indigo and Black

Indigo and black side-by-side points to a person whose spiritual advancement has been blocked, usually by a conservative religious upbringing. It can also reveal the presence of female sexual-healing energy within the person's sixth chakra, indicating that person's potential to offer long-distance or remote healing of another person's sexual energy.

### Gray and Black

Gray in combination with black indicates a person who is untrusting of yin, female energy. This is sometimes found in men who have been hurt by their mothers and have grown to mistrust female energy. Female energy makes them feel insecure.

## White

White, when appearing as extremely bright white or as crystal diamond white, represents the highest and most healing energy available. It is the white that lies at the core of all our chakras. It is the energy of our state of enlightenment, always present within each and every one of us, but hidden under seven encircling layers of rainbow-colored energy. It is the white of God. In terms of yin and yang, white also represents yang, male energy.

When healing a client using energy work in my massage practice, I sometimes see the color white. From personal experience I have learned to interpret this as meaning that no more healing work needs to be done on the part of the person's body I have been working on; the area is now clean and clear. White, in this respect, may be interpreted as "healed." There are different shades of this white energy, which may reflect different degrees of being healed:

> Plain white = healed
> Cream = almost healed
> Gray white = needs more healing

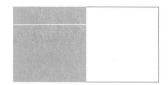

### Sky Blue and White

Sometimes during spiritual healing, the color combination of sky blue and white appears. This indicates the presence of the energy of Our Lady and is a very powerful healing energy to use. Although powerful, it is very yin and soft in the way it heals hurt energy, unlike ultraviolet or diamond white, which can be very yang and forceful in their effect.

## Gray

Gray is the color of the energy of insecurity. When you first connect with this energy in the body of a person, the first thing that happens is you get a strong feeling that you do not know what it is and you become insecure from not knowing what it is. This is the essence of insecurity. A person with a lot of this energy may be described as being a lost soul. When you are unclear about something in life or untrusting of something or someone, you generate gray energy in your subtle-energy body.

Metaphysically, the energy of insecurity is incredibly sticky. When you connect with it in the body of a person it rushes onto your hands and arms and sticks there and is really difficult to shake off. If you take on the energy of your client's insecurity early on in a massage, you will have to stop the massage and clean the energy from your hands, as to continue would mean putting the energy of insecurity back into the energy system of your client, doing them no good. You need to clean yourself of the gray energy completely, through whatever method of grounding or cleansing you use in your practice; for example, placing your hands over a candle flame until you feel all the stickiness burn off.

### Light or Pale Gray

This color reveals the presence of the emotional energies of grief or lightly experienced loneliness. It feels soft, spongy, and coldish when you sense it in the body of a person. When you hold the energy of grief in your own body, it metaphorically feels like gray clouds or gray cotton wool. This energy is often found in the body between upper breast and clavicle.

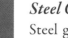

### Steel Gray

Steel gray is the color of the energy of tiredness, often chronic tiredness. When you connect with this energy in the body of another person, it can leave you feeling very tired. Metaphysically, the energy is neither heavy nor sticky; it simply makes you feel tired. It is different from other forms of gray energy in that it always has a metallic look or feel.

### Deep or Dark Gray

Dark gray reveals the presence of the energy of a mental disturbance, such as depression. Metaphysically it feels very heavy, and if you work with a person in massage to help release this energy it can leave you feeling heavy and very tired afterward. As a therapist, you need to be in strong physical and emotional condition when working with this energy. You also need to give yourself sufficient time to fully recover postmassage after working with this energy.

### Dark Steel Gray

Dark steel gray is the energy of cult—the energy that forms a cult and that holds a cult together. Metaphysically this color feels very heavy and is very difficult to pull out of a person. Although I describe this energy as deep steel gray, it does not have a metallic sheen to it. It is dull and flat in appearance, similar to brushed graphite. It is a very difficult energy to release from a massage client because cult energy, by its very nature, is a very powerful energy force. As a healer or massage therapist, your own energy levels need to be very robust when dealing with a client holding the energy of cult in their system.

The energy of cult is passed between individuals, most typically from teacher to student. It can also be transferred through the intellectual or corrupted spiritual teachings of the cult, through books, videos, lectures, or rituals. Additionally, cult energy is transferred through sexual connection between cult teacher/leader and student. The three chakras normally affected by cult energy are the sixth chakra, where the energy of spiritual wisdom is housed; the third chakra, where intellectual and academic energy is stored; and the second chakra, where our sexual energy is stored. Cult energy will adversely affect any or all of these areas of the body, making them heavy, cold, and contracted. If you are the child of a cult member, your red energy center, your first chakra, will be similarly affected.

In healing a person of the energy of cult, you have to work to strip out the dark steel gray color from the person's first, second, third, or sixth chakras, until whichever affected chakra is completely free of the color. This can be hard work, as energetically you are opposing the energy of the will of the cult leader, which is why, as a healer or therapist, your own energy levels need to be so robust.

## Brown

Like gray, there is nothing healthy about brown energy. In general, brown and shades of brown reveal weakness in one form or another.

Brown is the color of a self-belief held within the conscious mind, the third chakra, that keeps a person in a state of weakness or powerlessness. A classic example is the belief that you are not strong enough to get something done. This is a brown belief. Its color is a combination of yellow, a positive mental belief, and black, a negatively impacting energy, such as fear. Brown energy is usually found in the third chakra and in the TCM meridians associated with the third chakra: the spleen, stomach, liver, and gallbladder meridians.

### *Golden Brown or Honey Brown*
Honey brown is the color of the energy of words of anger that have not been expressed. Unexpressed anger is by its very nature a blockage in the flow of energy.

### Dark Brown

Dark brown is the energy of words that were formed but were not spoken. It is the energy of dead words, so it is dead energy. As a dead energy it causes deep blockage and can be very hard to release from the subtle-energy body. It is like trying to shift a dead weight. Unspoken words can be both positive or negative. Surprisingly, unused positive words, such as never telling someone you loved them while you had the chance to do so, can cause a blockage in your energy system. Words are very powerful forms of energy and should always be allowed to be freely expressed. Unspoken, or unused words, whether words of anger or love, cause energy blockage and a certain amount of physical discomfort. Dark brown energy is also very dry in its feel when you connect to it.

## Three-Color
## Energy Blockage Combinations

Sometimes energy blockages are revealed as a combination of three side-by-side colors. These are the most complex and difficult color combinations to interpret, yet they can reveal extremely accurate information. It is not within the scope of this book to discuss three-color combinations, simply because of their complexity and the sheer number of variations, but I will offer one example that I have come across frequently in my work: red, black, and orange.

In this example, red relates to family, black reveals pain, and orange means second chakra. This reveals a person whose second-chakra energy has been hurt by a family member.

## Therapist Burnout

Burnout is not uncommon in yoga or massage. It happens to teachers and therapists alike. There is the obvious cause of burnout—overworking—but there is also a subtle reason for burnout, which is related to mismatched energy and energy blockage caused by unfulfilled, subconscious needs.

For many years the reason why I taught Thai massage, the energy that drove me to teach, came from an unfulfilled subconscious need: the need to be heard. It was a need that extended all the way back into my early childhood, when my parents didn't listen to me. When teaching, I was happy when the class listened to what I had to say, but I felt lost and deeply insecure when they didn't. My need to be heard guaranteed a great class for students, as I made very sure it was interesting enough to get everybody listening, but I was not free in my teaching. I wasn't teaching for the simple pleasure of teaching; I was teaching in order to be heard. This is a mismatch of energy exchange: giving yellow energy in the expectation of receiving sky blue in return. A mismatched energy exchange can never properly fill the void left by the original unfulfilled energy. Having my students listen to me was not a substitute for my parents listening to me.

I know of some yoga teachers who teach in order to be respected by their students, and I know of massage therapists who massage in order to be loved by their clients. As long as the energies of love and respect flow in, the energies of massage and teaching flow out. It is when the cycle of this energy flow is broken, when the energies of love or respect stop flowing in, that problems arise. There is nothing coming in after everything has been given out. Result: collapse and burnout.

It is our unfulfilled subconscious energetic needs that are the hidden causes of burnout. If you are a teacher or therapist who regularly suffers burnout, you may have to look at yourself very honestly and ask: Why am I teaching yoga? Why am I giving massage? What need am I seeking to fulfill through my work? When do I suffer burnout?

What happens in class or in massage before burnout? What do I stop getting? What is the trigger?

Love from clients does not replace missing love from parents. Parental love is rooted in the first chakra. It is red energy. Love from clients comes into the body through the third chakra. It is yellow energy. As forms of love energy, they are totally mismatched. They may feel the same, but they're not. One is red, the other yellow. One is incapable of replacing or fulfilling the other. The belief in the opposite is an endless trap that goes round and round. This is the reason why some massage therapists need to keep the cycle of love energy coming in all the time, and why they collapse when the cycle breaks. If love from a client did replace unfulfilled love from a parent, then your energetic needs would be fulfilled and you would not collapse when the cycle breaks.

# Releasing Blockages
# in the Body

## 30 Energetic Ailment Indicators

This chapter describes thirty areas of the body where common energy blockages manifest as physical discomfort or pain, starting at the bottom of the body and working up, ending at the crown chakra. These energy blockages can be the result of one's upbringing, environment, family and friends, or current lifestyle. The origin and cause of each of the energy blockages is given, along with a physical description—what it feels like—and advice on how best to move through or release the blockage.

This illustrates how a range of physical conditions that present in the body, such as weakness in the knees, tightness in the hamstrings, or inflammation in the neck, can be part of a broader, underlying condition of energy blockage, oftentimes with roots that extend far back. As well, it shows that treating certain physical conditions at the point where they manifest, without reference to the energetic origin of the condition, is an incomplete approach—for example, treating the condition of tight shoulders by massaging the shoulder area, without referring to the energetic origin of tight shoulders, which is found in either the upper chest or at the rear of the solar plexus. We also find that oftentimes treatment for some physical conditions may involve an alteration in some aspect of one's lifestyle, mindset, or belief system that is contributing to the manifestation of the problem.

At all times the physical body is a mirror of the condition of the mind, whether it's the conscious, subconscious, or unconscious mind. The more rigid, tight, and unyielding the mind, the more rigid, tight, and unyielding the physical body (tight shoulders, neck, chest, abdomen, hips, hamstrings, psoas, ankles, etc.—the list is almost endless). The more free the mind, the more open, soft, warm, light, and loose the body is. However, do not confuse flexibility with softness. In terms of physical flexibility, you can have a longtime yoga practitioner capable of advanced asanas, yet when you massage this person he or she feels tense and tight. Flexibility does not necessarily mean openness.

Generally speaking, when massaging a client, if you find them to be overall warm, soft, and yielding, it is an excellent sign of good health and that they are on the right path in life. On the other hand, flexibility can often mean the client has simply found a way of hiding their issues and pains more deeply—more likely if the flexible person shows a degree of tenseness or tightness.

Though the following information is geared mainly toward massage therapists, others involved in energy practices, including yoga teachers and students, martial arts practitioners, and experienced meditators—basically, anyone who is on the path of self-realization—will also find this information insightful. To help illustrate this, some of the ailment descriptions refer to how the ailment feels in the body of a massage client, while other descriptions refer to how the ailment feels in your own body. Sometimes, if you have been holding an ailment in your own body for a long time, you lose the sensitivity necessary to feel it in yourself and so you need a fresh pair of hands, those of a therapist, to point it out to you. This is why the "How it feels in the body of a massage client" is also useful to read when attempting to form a self-diagnosis.

As my own background is in Thai massage, a form of massage that takes place on a massage mat on the floor similar to a shiatsu treatment, some of the references given in treatment advice, such as lifting a client's leg off the ground, refer to massage given on the floor but can be adjusted for table massage too. Please be aware also that a degree of difficulty arises in the description of the exact location of some of the ailments. This is because the ailments being described are ailments of the subtle energy body and not of the physical body and as such have no corresponding traditional Western anatomical location. In energy work or energy healing, *energy* is the anatomy.

## 30 COMMON ENERGY BLOCKAGES

1. Tight Ankles
2. Weak Knees
3. Tight Quadriceps
4. Tightness along the Outside of the Thigh
5. Tight Hamstrings
6. Tight AIIS
7. Tightness in the Inside of the Thigh
8. Tightness at the Tops of the Adductor Magnus and Gracilis Muscles
9. Tight or Closed Hips
10. Compression below the Sacroiliac Joint
11. Weakness or Pain at the Top of the Sacrum
12. Asymmetry
13. Pain in the Outside of the Hip
14. Tight Psoas
15. Weak Lower Back
16. Tightness in the Midback
17. Tightness between the Shoulder Blades
18. Stiffness in the Area of the Shoulder Blades
19. Pain in the Center or Bottom Edge of the Scapula
20. Upper-Arm Pain
21. Pain or Weakness inside the Elbow
22. Forearm Tightness
23. Weak Wrists
24. Pain in the Right Arm
25. Coldness between the Upper Chest and the Clavicle
26. Pain in the Trapezius
27. Inflammation at the Sides of the Neck
28. Tightness at the Back of the Neck
29. Ears, Head, and Neck Pain
30. The Crown

A certain amount of caution must be exercised in using the information provided here. The description of each condition and its underlying cause should be used first and foremost as a method of self-diagnosis, an aid to help you better understand what is going on in your own body. Although you may find any of these blockages in the body of a massage client or a yoga student, to use this information as a diagnostic tool on another person is something that should only be undertaken with great sensitivity and awareness. You cannot say to a client or student with closed hips, "This reveals you are closed to life." This is both inappropriate and irresponsible. Where this information *is* valuable in the context of a massage treatment or yoga class, if you are a therapist or teacher, is in the ways it suggests an empathetic approach to understanding the deeper, underlying causes of many common problems, many of which we all suffer from at one time or another.

## 1. Tight Ankles

Tightness in the ankle extension reveals a blockage in the stomach meridian at the ST 41 acupuncture point at the top of the dorsum of the foot. In Thai massage, this point is known as the KHC point (knee pain, headache, and cramp). This reveals an overall imbalance in the quality of energy running in the stomach meridian, and it is this imbalance that causes the blockage and its resulting physical manifestation: tightness. The origin of this blockage lies behind the nipple on the same side of the body as the ankle in question. The blockage is in the heart, or fourth chakra, which may be deficient in the fire energy of love or the water energy of play but excessive in the air energy of material wealth or intellectual provision. The effect of excessive air energy in any part of the body is to cause tension, tightness, or hardness in that part of the body. Tightness in the ankle extension usually indicates a person who has not experienced enough love or play in their lives, yet has been sufficiently provided for educationally and financially.

In general, tightness in the ankle extension is mirrored by tightness in the front of the knee, also reflecting insufficient love and play (see number 2 in this chapter), and tightness in the AIIS, reflecting anger at

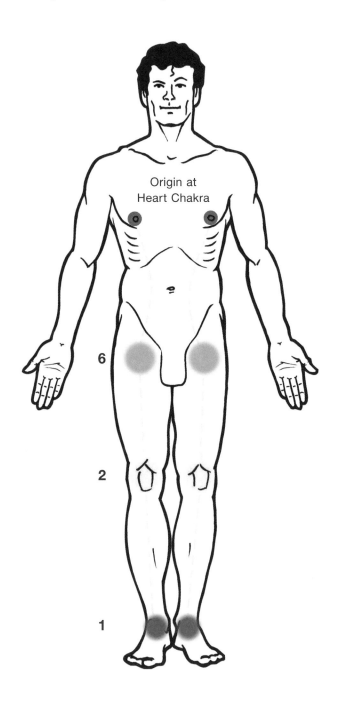

*Fig. 8.1. Tight ankles (1), weak knees (2), and tight AIIS (6)*

not having sufficient love and play (see number 6 in this chapter). The origin of the blockage, behind the nipple, is the location of the pain of the heart at being insufficiently loved. All points of tightness are on the stomach meridian, the meridian that energetically connects the heart with the feet. When the heart is closed, the ankle is usually similarly closed. See figure 8.1.

**What it feels like in the body of a massage client:** Lying in supine position, the client is unable to extend foot. There is very little or no plantar flexion. It feels as if the foot is being held at a 90 degree angle to the horizontal. The energy holding the foot in this position can be found in the shallow indentation between the bottom of the tibia and the top of the foot, between stomach meridian points 41 and 42.

**Treatment:** In the treatment of tight ankles, as well as massaging the ankle area itself, additional attention should be given to the front of the knee, the AIIS, and the region of the heart. As tightness in the ankles is caused by an insufficiency in the energy of love or play, it works best if you treat these other body areas with love, fire energy, or with a sense of playfulness, water energy.

## 2. Weak Knees

In general, weakness in the knees reflects a deficiency in either water energy or fire energy running through the knee. A deficiency in water energy reflects a lack of fun, play, or support in your life, or not believing in yourself. A deficiency in fire energy reflects a lack of love or self-love. There are two types of knee weakness: weakness in the front of the knee and weakness at the back of the knee.

### Front of the Knee
Weakness in the front of the knee reflects an excess of air energy in the knee and a deficiency in fire and water energies. This means that

your environment, past or present, may have sufficiently provided for you financially and educationally, but insufficiently provided you with love and fun or play. The air energy is housed on the stomach meridian, which runs through the front of the knee. Weakness in the front of the right knee relates to insufficient love, emotion, play, and fun shared between you and your father's side of the family. It may also indicate a lack of self-love in your father. Weakness in the front of the left knee relates to insufficient love, play, and fun shared between you and your mother's side of the family. It may also indicate your mother's lack of love for herself. See figure 8.1, page 242.

**What it feels like in the body of a massage client:** The kneecap feels cold; the kneecap bone may also feel empty.

**Treatment:** Cup the area of the kneecap with your hands, bringing the warmth of loving intention to the area. Alternatively, cup the area and play with it, giving rise to the water energy of fun and applying it to this body area. In massage, use soft, gentle energy. Strong or vigorous technique is a use of air energy, which causes further imbalance to the already excessive presence of air energy in the kneecap area. Weakness in the front of the knee indicates tightness in the stomach meridian running through the knee, which is linked to tightness in the AIIS and along the stomach meridian running up the front of the body to a point under the clavicle. Proper treatment for weakness in the front of the knee may therefore require additional treatment around the AIIS and along the stomach meridian.

## *Back of the Knee*

Insufficient heat in the water energy running through the back of the knee housed in the kidney meridian running inside the medial knee ligament reflects a lack of support in your life or a lack of belief in yourself. As well, knees carry the weight of another person's expectations of you, specifically, one or both of your parents. In many cases, a parent's expectation of you to succeed in life can be due to their own weakness in not being able to achieve or succeed in their life, thus the energy that is passed on to you at the time of conception is the energy of weakness. It is this energy of weakness, disguised as expectation, that can cause the knees to be weak. Often the two are connected. Weakness in the back of right knee indicates a lack of support or lack of belief in you from your father's side of the family. If you are female, it may also refer to your husband's lack of support or belief in you. Weakness in the back of the left knee indicates a lack of support or lack of belief in you from your mother's side of the family. If you are male, it may also refer to your wife's lack of support or belief in you.

**What it feels like in the body of a massage client:** The back of the knee is cold and the area feels dense when you press your thumb into it.

**Treatment:** As the weakness reveals a lack of support, just before you commence massaging the area, lift the entire knee and lower leg off the ground and hold them close to you. It is important to hold the client's foot off the ground too, as they feel that the ground underfoot is not providing them with sufficient support. Give the feeling to your client that you are holding and supporting them fully. It is the energy of your support that brings the healing to the back of your client's knee.

## 3. Tight Quadriceps

The condition of the quadriceps reflects the energetic connection between you and your ancestors. Tightness reflects the absence of openness in communication, emotion, love, and support. Tightness in the right quadriceps indicates that the lack is between you and your father, and indicates the tension that exists between your father and his family. The tenser these relationships are, the tighter the center of the quadriceps. The left quadriceps corresponds to your mother and your mother's side of the family. The main knot of tightness is on the stomach meridian, the meridian of inheritance. See figure 8.2, page 246.

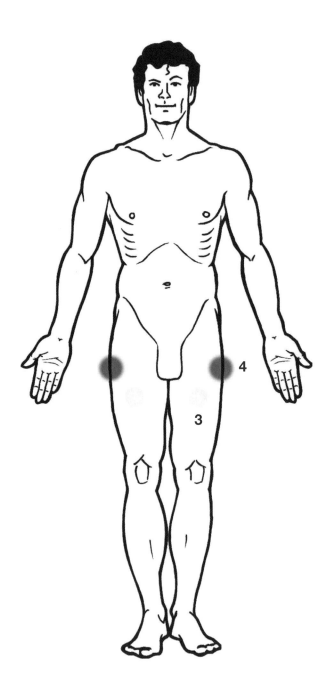

Fig. 8.2. Tightness in the quadriceps (3) and
along the outside of the thighs (4)

**What it feels like in the body of a massage client:** A small knot in the muscle in the front center of the quadriceps that feels a little like the top of a finger knuckle. The location loosely corresponds to the location of stomach meridian point 32.

**Treatment:** Place the center of the palm of one of your hands directly on the muscle knot. Gently clasp the surrounding area with your fingers and thumb. Hold the grip, allowing the heat from your palm to work into the knot. Gently massage the area, but without breaking your grip. At the center of your palm is a small energy center, or minor chakra, which is linked to the energy of your heart. So in holding your client's quadriceps in this manner, you are imparting the warming energy of your heart to your client and it is this warming energy that will help release the knot in the muscle, caused by insufficient love, or fire energy, running through the stomach meridian on this point.

## 4. Tightness along the Outside of the Thigh

This tightness runs along the gallbladder meridian, or in Thai massage the Thai Sen Kalathari, on the outside of the upper leg. This is the area of the body around which you wear your metaphysical body armor. It is the energy you use in your defense against letting others in, against revealing the truth about yourself and all you have done—your needs, feelings, and emotions. Defending against letting others in is the behavior of self-control shaped by a belief that something unfavorable will happen to you if you reveal your innermost and deepest self. For example, if you have an opinion that goes against the majority opinion, you may believe that by offering it you will be judged negatively by others. This belief is further complicated by emotions such as fear, shame, humiliation, guilt, etc. This is why this blockage or tightness in the outer thigh can be difficult to release, as it is being held in place by two types of subtle energy: mental and emotional. Sometimes this body armor is not wholly your own body armor, but that of a parent who may have never revealed him- or herself fully, and who then passed the energy of their defense against letting others in into your body at the time of conception. See figure 8.2, page 246.

**What it feels like in the body of a massage client:** The space running between the rectus femoris and vastus lateralis muscles will feel tight and slightly cold, causing both muscles, close to the running of this space, to additionally feel tight and slightly cold.

**Treatment:** This area of tightness extends to the outside of the greater trochanter. From there it travels through the pelvic girdle, close to the running of the gallbladder meridian, to the sacroiliac joint, where its origin lies. Therefore, in treatment, the whole area requires massage. Massage technique may require a mixture of vigorous and gentle touch; you have to play around with it to find out. Some people's energy is suited to vigorous massage, others suited to a more gentle approach. Be guided by how soft your chosen approach makes the muscles feel.

# 5. Tight Hamstrings

The energetic origin of tight hamstrings is a small but very deep and severely icy cold area of energy between the sit bone, the ischial tuberosity, and the inside of the top of the femur. It is in TCM, Urinary Bladder point UB 36. Tight hamstrings indicate the energy of abandonment in infancy and/or the energy of loneliness in early childhood. The cold energy is related to all the times when as a baby you wanted to be with your mother and father but they weren't available. Maybe they regularly put you into another room, or maybe they were absent for long periods of time. Either way, as an infant you experienced this as abandonment, and you were unable to crawl to or otherwise find your parents so you were forced to sit in the painful energy of your own loneliness, which as an adult has gathered close to your sit bones. See figure 8.3.

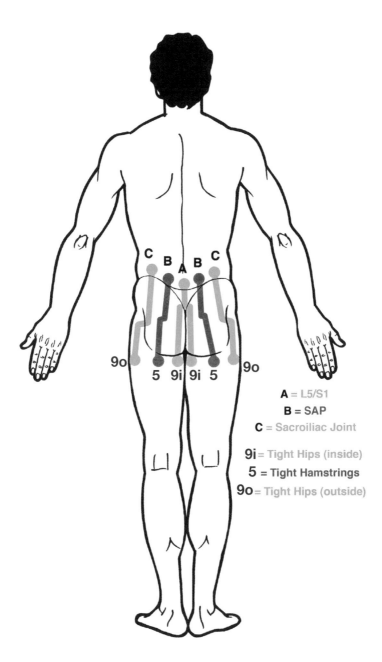

*Fig. 8.3. Tight hamstrings (5) and tight hips (9)*

**What it feels like in your body and in the body of a massage client:** A contracted, tight hamstring muscle is generally dense, heavy, and coldish. Closer to the bone, the ligament feels very tight. Although the hamstring muscle and tendon feel tight, both are actually in a state of contraction, caused by very cold energy.

**Treatment:** The area of contraction ascends to either side of the base of the first chakra, the perineum, and runs very close along the tailbone up to the space between L5 and S1. The whole area requires treatment. As with tightness on the outside of the thigh, treatment may be either vigorous, gentle, or a mixture of both. It can also be beneficial to work in the heart area of the client in order to generate the heating energy of love and self-love from within the heart chakra, and to use this warming energy to balance the cold energy of loneliness or abandonment. In terms of energy work and the chakras, the heart chakra, the fourth chakra, is energetically linked to the root chakra, the first chakra. When the warming heat of love is generated in the heart chakra, a warming heat is also spontaneously released into the root chakra, helping to melt the cold energy of loneliness and abandonment in the base of the root chakra and at the top of the femur.

# 6. Tight AIIS

Tightness in the AIIS, the anterior inferior iliac spine, the bony eminence on the anterior border of the hip bone, indicates the energy of anger at being abandoned in infancy. This relates to the times when as a baby you wanted the love and support of a parent but didn't receive it, which created anger in you. As an infant, you were unable to do anything to escape this anger, and so you were left to sit in its energy. As an adult, this energy has accumulated in the front of your AIIS, causing a blockage in the stomach meridian linking the heart with the foot. It is this energy blockage—the presence of anger at being unloved—

that blocks the flow of love in the stomach meridian. As with tightness on the outside of the thigh, sometimes this energy blockage may additionally contain a degree of ancestral energy, i.e., the energy of your parent's anger at being abandoned by their parents. See figure 8.1, page 242.

**What it feels like in the body of a massage client:** When you place your hand flat on the AIIS, the surrounding area feels dense or semihard.

**Treatment:** Caution is required when treating this area in massage. Do not use thumb acupressure. Releasing AIIS energy causes a feverlike condition. Fever is the release of strongly felt energy, usually anger. It causes the heart to race and the pulse to quicken. It also makes you feel hot, although your actual body temperature doesn't change. Place the palm of your hand on the area and use its heat and natural weight to do the work. Do not overwork this area.

## 7. Tightness in the Inside of the Thigh (Liver Meridian, Iliopsoas/ Adductor Muscles)

This condition indicates anger at being unloved and is energetically linked to tightness in the adductor magnus and gracilis muscles (liver meridian) and the AIIS (stomach meridian). All three ailments are linked in that they reside in the body area governed by the first chakra and relate to the connection between child and parents during infancy. Anger is a yellow energy. Childhood anger is housed in the yellow layer of the first chakra and is distributed around the area of the body governed by the first chakra on two of the meridians associated with yellow energy: the stomach and liver meridians. See figure 8.4, page 252.

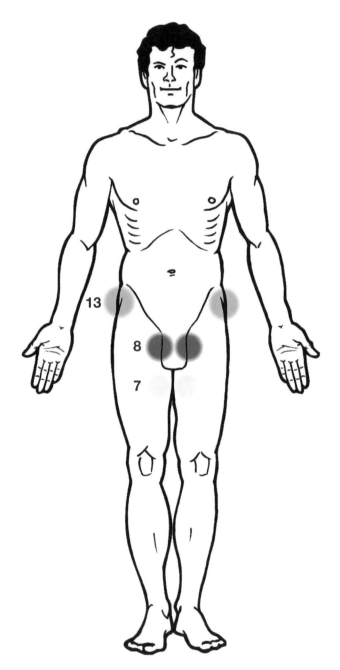

*Fig. 8.4. Tight inner thigh (7), tight adductor magnus and gracilis (8),
and pain in the outer hip (13)*

**What it feels like in your body and in the body of a massage client:** This can be a very sensitive area to touch and can be quite itchy or ticklish too. On deeper touch, the feeling is of a subtle to strong denseness around the running of the liver meridian or the Thai Sen Kalathari on the inside of the upper leg.

**Treatment:** The condition requires a regular massage workout. Do not dwell overlong here, however, as this area is often sensitive. Overworking the area can eventually stir up the energy of anger and may get your client angry at you. Support with gentle work on the AIIS.

## 8. Tightness at the Tops of the Adductor Magnus and Gracilis Muscles Close to the Perineum

Tightness in this area of the upper thigh indicates a mistrust of one of the sexes. Tightness on the right reveals mistrust of the male sex; on the left, mistrust of the female sex. This mistrust can come from either or both of two sources:

- During the earliest stage in life, between you and your parents. If the relationship between you and your mother was hurtful or loveless, it will cause you to mistrust the female sex. If it was between you and your father, it will lead to your mistrust of the male sex.
- The inherited energy of mistrust between your parents, up to the point of your conception and in the years following your birth

Mistrust can be the result of being hurt by someone, or of living with someone who never reveals themselves to you. In the latter case, you end up living with someone you do not know, someone you cannot trust. In adulthood, mistrust that is rooted in childhood may not be present on the surface, but it can arise after being in a relationship for a few years. See figure 8.4.

**What it feels like in your body and in the body of a massage client:** The muscles are so tight that they feel like lengths of steel rope extending outward from the perineum.

**Treatment:** This is an area not easily treated in massage, nor is it recommended to do so, as the area lies so close to the external genitalia. The release of this condition takes many years of self-healing and is linked to the healing of the first chakra, early childhood and ancestry, the third chakra, the seat of anger, and the fourth chakra, the seat of love. If you are very sensitive to the energies in your body and if you have been doing self-healing for many years, you may find the action of placing your hands on your solar plexus, the front of your third chakra, in an act of self-love loosens the adductor magnus and gracilis muscles.

# 9. Tight or Closed Hips

Open or closed/tight hips reflect the degree of openness or closedness you have toward life. This openness or closedness occurs as a result of the relationship between you and your parents from the time of your conception until you were about two or three years of age. If the relationship was open and warm, your hips will tend to be similarly open; if the relationship was cold and closed, your hips will be similarly closed. If you had a difficult relationship with your father but an open one with your mother, your right hip will be more closed. If the cold relationship was with your mother, then your left hip will be more closed. The origin of the energy that causes hips to close and hamstrings to tighten is the navel. From the navel, this energy travels through the torso to the base of the lumbar spine between L5 and S1. From there it spreads outward, through the superior articular process (SAP) to the sacroiliac joint. From there it travels downward through the pelvic girdle to the insides/outsides and front/back of the top of the femur. This is why the hips can be held tight from the inside of the femur or from the outside of the femur, or both inside and outside simultaneously. See figure 8.3, page 249.

**What it feels like in your body:** When you try to sit in either quarter, half, or full lotus, you find that one or both of your knees do not touch the floor.

**Treatment:** In every case, the area of treatment for closed hips or tight hamstrings is on either side of the spine between L3 and S1 and across the buttocks between the sit bones and the greater trochanter. The whole area needs to be massaged and the quality of the energy in your touch needs to be a loving one, as the energetic reason for hips being closed is a lack of love.

## 10. Compression below the Sacroiliac Joint

Hips can also be blocked from opening by the presence of compressed energy below the sacroiliac joint, in the soft buttock area between the sit bone and the top of the femur, in the area known in Thai massage as "the boomerang." The origination point of this energy block is at the rear of the third chakra, on both sides of the spine, in the area around L1 and L2. This is the compressed energy of two subtly different things:

- The emotional energy of the fear of what will happen if you fully commit to something and it doesn't work out
- The mental energy of the belief that if you give yourself fully to something you will fail, for instance, on setting up your own business

Both energies feed each other, and although they may appear the same they are not. One energy is emotional, the other mental. Yet both are energy blockages. This blockage reveals a deeper lack of trust in life, extending back to the time when, as an infant, you gave yourself fully to either or both your parents, but they did not meet your needs. Tightness in the area of the hips and pelvic girdle is related to not being sufficiently loved in infancy. As an infant, this early experience taught you that you will be hurt if you leave yourself open, so you close up in order to protect yourself. Part of this closing is the closing of your hips. It is a purely defensive and protective action.

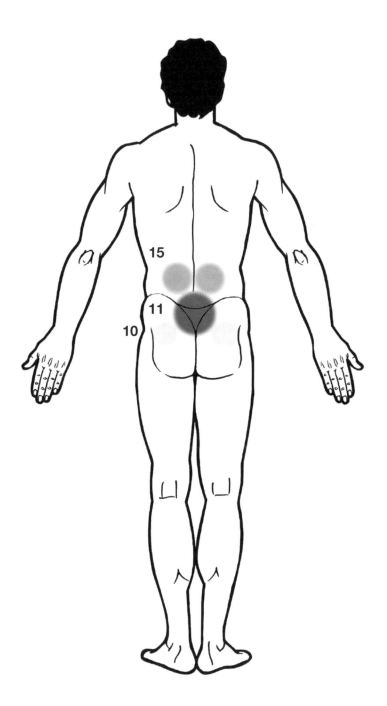

*Fig. 8.5. Compression below the SI joint (10), weakness at the top of the sacrum (11), and weak lower back (15)*

As mentioned at the outset of this chapter, guard against using the cause of tight hips as some sort of judgment. If you suffer from tight hips yourself, the chances are extremely high that your parents also suffered the same circumstances in childhood, and sometimes the energy of your parents' unhappiness gets passed on to your energy system at the time of your conception. And yes, you too will pass along these tendencies to your own children—it's all part of the cycle of life. No one is to blame. The important thing to note is that you can break the cycle. See figure 8.5.

**What it feels like in your body:** When in massage, lying on your side, the therapist presses their thumb into the soft area of your buttock and you feel an immediate, intense pain.

**Treatment:** Massage the whole area between LI to L5, crossing to the sacroiliac joint and downward across the soft area of the buttock onto the outside of the thigh. This will have a healing effect on the energies of belief (from the third chakra) and fear (from the second chakra). As the issues of love, support, and trust are at the heart of the symptoms of closed hips, you should address this in your treatment. Work lovingly and slowly in the area. Create feelings of trust and support. Try not to create unnecessary pain with a vigorous massage technique.

## 11. Weakness or Pain at the Top of the Sacrum

The top of the sacrum, on either side of the spine between L5 and S1, is the site of one of the major pains and weaknesses released when one undertakes more advanced self-development, whether through yoga, meditation, martial arts, etc. This area of the body stores a specific type of energy that creates weakness. Although this energy is inherent in all of us, it is only released by the person involved in self-developmental work. It is an energy that is dark gray in color and when released causes acute physical weakness and pain. The pain and weakness makes it extremely difficult to lift your leg off the ground or to bend downward or forward to any extent. In extreme cases you become unable to walk or get out of bed. Upon the release of this blocked energy, the concepts of pain and weakness enter your consciousness, making them real, felt pain. This is the point of the hidden energy in this part of your body: to give credence to the concepts of pain and weakness. This pain often begins to gently release over a period of years, causing only minor intermittent inconvenience until a trigger event, which causes the full release. The trigger event is usually an everyday, mundane event, such as stepping into or out of the shower. See figure 8.5, page 256.

**What it feels like in your body:** A catastrophic release of pain and loss of muscular power in your lower back.

**Treatment:** This acute condition can last several days or weeks, so it is advised to seek professional medical help as soon as the release kicks in, as the pain experienced will force you to move your body in a way to compensate for the pain, creating additional pain and tension in other muscles. A visit to a chiropractor practicing one of the more gentle forms of chiropractic, such as McTimoney chiropractic, is highly recommended. Gentle exercising, such as walking in a straight line on a level surface, alternative knee raises while lying in a supine position, or gentle yogic cobra asana all help in rehabilitation.

# 12. Asymmetry

The internal feeling of asymmetry between the left-hand side and right-hand side of your body reveals that your internal female side is not communicating with your internal male side. This is reflective of certain female figures in your life not communicating with certain male figures in your life, such as your mother not communicating with your father, your grandfather not communicating with your grandmother, you not talking to your mother/father, you not talking to your sister/brother, or you not talking to your partner/spouse. The greater the block in the communication between the female and male side of your family, the greater the feeling of asymmetry in your own body. As this is an overall bodily sensation, it cannot be shown as manifesting in a particular location in the body.

**What it feels like in your body:** The feeling, during regular yoga practice, that the left-hand side of your torso reacts very differently in asana than the right-hand side of your torso.

**Treatment:** In massage, on the back of the body you will find a very narrow band of tightness running right along the spine on both sides. This needs to be softened and released. Additionally massage laterally across the spine between the vertebrae to move energy across and through the spine. On the front of the body, gentle lateral massage across the body in sweeping infinity moves (like a horizontal 8) with the midpoint of the move crossing on the center line of the body. Work across the heart, solar plexus, and lower abdominal regions.

## 13. Pain in the Outside of the Hip

Pain in the outside of the hip that has nothing to do with any tightness in the hips relates to the energetic connections to your siblings and/or spouse. If your brother or husband has caused you pain in life, the energetic connection you have to him will manifest as pain in your right hip. The energy of this pain spreads down through the leg, creating physical leg pain and difficulty in walking. The energetic connection to a sister or wife is in the left hip. See figure 8.4, page 252.

**What it feels like in the body of a massage client:** When you place your hand across your client's iliac crest, you will feel an area of cold on the center of your palm. If you are sensitive to the colors of energy, you will see the condition as an area of black energy on the outside of the iliac crest.

**Treatment:** Massage the whole area from the iliac crest down the outside of the thigh and lower leg to the foot. If you are sensitive to the energetic color of the ailment, symbolically grab and pull the blob of black energy off the iliac crest.

# 14. Tight Psoas

Tightness or rigidity in the area of the psoas (psoas major and iliacus muscles) reflects rigidity in lifestyle, such as a lifestyle built on structure and routine or the rigidity with which you judge life, for example, that life is unfair, or the rigidity with which you judge others, for example, "My boss is a total bastard." The degree of tightness in the psoas reflects the degree of rigidity you impose on your lifestyle or the degree of rigidity with which you hold on to your beliefs. The energy used in holding on to routine and rigid belief and judgment is third-chakra energy, energy of the air element. Air energy causes muscles to tense, tighten, and harden. The more you hold to your rigid lifestyle and beliefs, the more air energy you use and hold in your body, and therefore the more rigidity you experience in your psoas. If the types of beliefs you hold on to are painful, such as "life is hard" or "nobody loves me" or "I am a victim," it follows that you metaphysically hold on to pain, which then manifests in the psoas.

Pain in the psoas can also reflect the pain of having to conform to a life of structure and routine, the fear of feeling or becoming lost without structure and routine, or the despair that comes later in life from realizing that seeking solace through structure and routine, and rigidity in general, does not provide the hoped-for comfort. As this condition lies within the body area governed by the first chakra, there may be some ancestral influence in this condition. Check for structured, routine-driven lifestyles in your recent ancestry. People use structure and routine in life to fill the void left by an absence of love.

Paradoxically, students who try to use yoga to release the psoas may find it difficult to do so, as using yoga to create a specific outcome is a form of structured, rigid behavior. Using a structured approach to release a condition caused by the use of structure is counterproductive. You cannot exert control over a part of your body in order to set it free. You have to allow your body to find its own freedom. This comes from surrendering to your yoga practice instead of trying to use it or control it for a specific outcome. See figure 8.6.

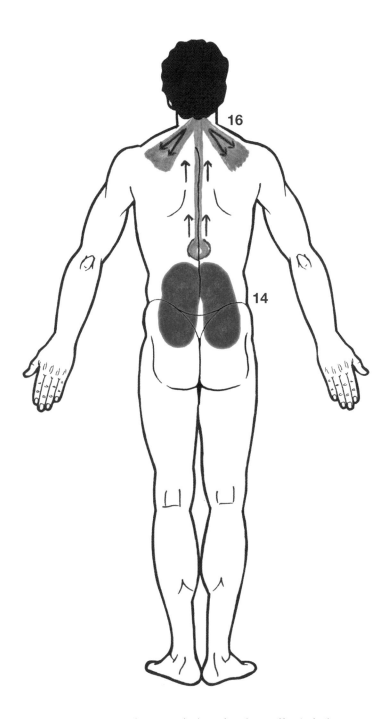

*Fig. 8.6. Tight psoas (14) and tight midback (16)*

**What it feels like in your body:** A dull pain that extends downward from either side of the navel toward the inside of the groin or toward the back of the top of the thigh. It always feels like it is deep inside, a core pain. Sympathetic to the running of the kidney and stomach meridians in this part of the body, the meridians that govern inherited patterns of behavior through ancestry.

**Treatment:** Here is a lovely, relaxing exercise for self-treatment to help release the psoas. Lie on your back and draw your feet toward your buttocks, keeping your knees pointing up toward the ceiling. Now rub your hands together until they are red hot and place them on both sides of your abdomen, just above the groin, with the ball of your hand resting on the ilium and your fingers pointing toward your central line. Just allow the heat from your hands to sink into this body area. The key to the exercise is to generate body heat in the lower abdominal region, close to the groin. Allow fifteen minutes for the exercise.

# 15. Weak Lower Back

A weak lower back between L4 and L3 is caused by kidney-energy imbalance or depletion, typically caused by any of the following: overworking, an overall feeling of timidity or fearfulness in life, telling lies and having to listen to lies, excessive pursuit of one or more pleasures, addiction, or wearing clothing that is too light during weather when the sun is hot but the air is cool or damp. See figure 8.5, page 256.

**What it feels like in your body and in the body of a massage client:** A feeling of tightness or weakness in the muscles on either side of the spine around L4 and L3, along with a slight swelling of the kidneys.

**Treatment:** Depleted kidneys respond very well to rest, correct nutrition, and warmth. The use of hot herbal compresses on this body area in massage can bring great relief, especially if warming herbs like ginger, turmeric, or garlic are used in the compress. Also, warm the soles of the feet under the second toe in the area corresponding to point I on the kidney meridian, according to the TCM classification. As well, a course in TCM will bring faster relief to kidney-energy depletion and lower-back weakness and is preferable to regular massage, which simply removes the tiredness from the muscles exhausted by the depletion of energy.

## 16. Tightness in the Midback

Tightness in the area between L2 and L1 is caused by a chronic or acute buildup of harmful emotional and mental energies related to stress, such as having to put up with a highly toxic work environment, trying to hold everything together, the fear and belief that everything will be lost if you do not hold everything together yourself, the regret at getting into the stressful situation in the first place and the feeling of powerlessness that results, and the enforced self-control and anger and frustration at having to put up with everything going on around you. It requires enormous amounts of energy to do, believe, feel, and hold on to all these things, and all these stressful energies build up inside the body, creating pressure, tension, agitation, shaking, clenching, tightness, and hardness. The place where all these energies originate, giving rise to stress, is the front of the solar plexus chakra. When the condition of stress is strong, the energy of stress spreads backward, from the front of the solar plexus, through the torso, to the back of the solar plexus, coming out of the midback in the space between the L2 and L1. From there the energy of stress forms a thin line of tension or tightness that runs very close to the running of the spine from the back of L2 to the back of the head. See figure 8.6, page 261.

**What it feels like in the body of a massage client:** The energy concentrated between L2 and LI travels upward along both sides of the spine to the base of the skull, and from there it fans downward into the shoulder area. As it does so, it creates hardness and tightness in the muscles. The energy of stress is the most common cause of tightness in the shoulders. When the pressure of stress energy is chronic, it rises up either side of the spine, continuing through the base of the skull, causing pressure and tension in the head, the physical manifestation of which is headache.

**Treatment:** When helping a client suffering from this kind of stress, all parts of the body carrying the energy of stress need to be addressed, not just the shoulders, which is where the client tends to feel the effects the most. In particular, work to release the thin line of tightness that runs very close to the running of the spine. This is the key line of tension to release. Don't worry if you find that you have to massage the area more than once in order to release the tension; this is normal.

# 17. Tightness between the Shoulder Blades

This small area of the body traversing the spine between the shoulder blades houses the energy of unforgivingness and judgment toward oneself and others. The more you hold on to unforgivingness and judgment, the tighter this area of the body will be. This kind of attitude toward life blocks the energy of the heart at the back of the heart chakra in the area between the shoulder blades. The heart desires its owner to be free, forgiving, loving, and nonjudgmental. See figure 8.7.

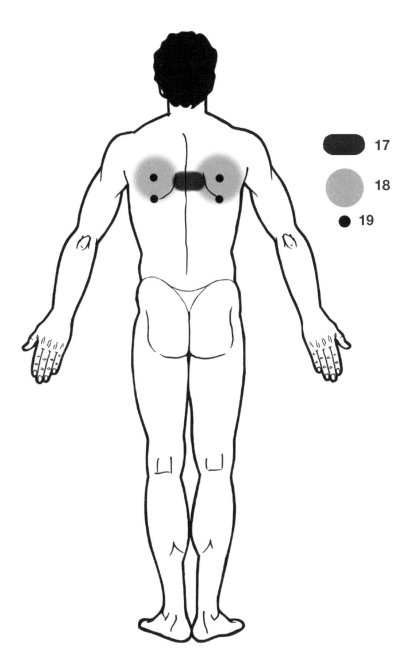

*Fig. 8.7. Tightness between the shoulder blades (17),
stiff shoulder blades (18), and pain in the scapula (19)*

**What it feels like in the body of a massage cleint:** A semihard "golf ball" of energy between the shoulder blades. The energy of unforgivingness additionally contracts the muscles around the shoulder blades and the tops of the arms and outer arms, causing pain in the running of the large intestine, small intestine, triple heater, and heart meridians in the upper arm.

**Treatment:** After massaging the area between the shoulder blades to reduce the physical tightness, work gently and energetically on the front of the heart chakra to build up warmth in this area. Hold the warmth there for as long as possible, allowing it to dissipate back into the heart chakra.

# 18. Stiffness in the Area of the Shoulder Blades

In general, the shoulder blades relate to the correct use or misuse of your life-force energy. The pain of not being able to discern what is good for you and what is not good for you in life or of not knowing how best to use the gifts you already have is held in the small intestine meridian, the exact point of pain coming from TCM point SI 11, in the center of the scapula. The scapula is the area of the body that lies between the energy of the small intestine meridian and spleen meridian, which governs life-force energy. When there is a blockage between these two meridians, as when these two meridians are not working together, a parallel physical blockage results, manifesting as stiffness.

Stiffness in the area of the shoulder blades usually reveals you are going in the wrong direction in life, or you are doing something in life that isn't serving your highest purpose. This is actually a positive and predictive pain, showing that you either need to make an adjustment in your life direction or that an important change is about to come into your life and you will have to adjust to align yourself to this new change or direction. This may involve letting go of some old ways of thinking and behaving and adapting to newer, higher ways of thinking and behaving. The change will take place when you become aligned, at which point the energy between the spleen and small intestine meridians will flow freely, removing the blockage between the two. It is the blockage of energy between the two meridians, found in the area of the shoulder blades, that causes the feeling of resistance and lack of mobility. See figure 8.7, page 265.

## Stiffness in the Area of the Left Shoulder Blade

Stiffness in the area of the left shoulder indicates you do not yet know what to do or what direction to take when it comes to using your energies or intuition in the highest and best way for you. This ailment only arises after you have awakened your higher, intuitive, spiritual energies.

Such pain can be witnessed in yoga practice when the time comes for the student to change the reason why they practice. Most people start yoga for a reason, such as wanting to be able touch their toes. This becomes their goal in yoga and they channel their life-force energy into their practice in order to achieve this goal. Sometimes, however, such a student can become interested in other aspects of yoga on their journey, such as discovering the yoga sutras of Patanjali. When such a student suddenly experiences left shoulder stiffness after months of practice, it is their shoulders telling them it is time to leave behind the goal of wanting to touch their toes and explore a potentially deeper goal in yoga. This is the spleen and small intestine meridians telling the student that widening their yoga practice to include additional study, such as of Patanjali, is a better use of their life-force energy than merely wanting to touch their toes. When the practitioner adjusts their practice to include study of Patanjali, the stiffness in the left shoulder disappears.

## Stiffness in the Area of the Right Shoulder Blade

Once you have established a general direction to take in life that is aligned with your higher energies, the question of how to specifically use your higher energies in the best way for yourself arises. If you are uncertain or blocked as to how to go about doing this, you might experience stiffness in the region of the right shoulder. For example, you have established that you are to be a teacher, but are now unsure as to how to use the energy of teaching in the most effective way, i.e., general schooling, special-needs education, or specialized one-subject teaching (e.g., art, movement, dance, drama, yoga, meditation, etc.). Don't worry too much about this pain. If you listen to it and surrender to it, the answer as to what to do will eventually come to you. Going through the experience of pain, however, is part of the process of listening to your body and surrendering to your higher self in guiding you through life.

**What it feels like in the body of a massage client:** There is a layer of dense, coldish sponginess covering the area of the shoulder blade.

**Treatment:** Three areas need addressing in massage treatment: the shoulder blades, the heart chakra, and the sixth chakra. First, massage the area of the shoulder blade(s) with very warm hands until the coldish quality in the spongy tissue dissipates. Now put your client in supine position. Massage and open the fronts of both the fourth and sixth chakras with gentle circular movements. Place one hand on the sixth chakra, with your other on the fourth, and with the power of intention move energy from the sixth to the fourth. This helps to bring the knowledge of the future into the present, where hopefully it will be felt in the heart, in the fourth chakra. If the treatment is successful, the client will be struck by an inspirational idea or thought about what to do in life a few days following the treatment. When this happens, the shoulder condition releases.

# 19. Pain in the Center or Bottom Edge of the Scapula

## *Pain in the Center of the Scapula*

Pain in the center of the scapula is caused by forcing your hands to do something they are not free to do or are not happy to do, for example, forcing yourself to paint or knit in order to escape feelings of loneliness. Here the freedom to create is subjugated by the need to create, which is determined by the need for escape. This is a misuse of the energy of creative expression and, by extension, a misuse of your hands to support such misuse. This enforced incorrect use of your life-force energy causes a blockage in the energy flowing between the spleen and small intestine meridians in the region of the scapula, the exact point of pain being TCM point SI 11. It is this blockage that gives rise to physical pain. Some massage therapists get this pain when it is time for them to stop their massage career, yet they do not stop because they do not know what else to do. Continuing to massage when your heart or your intuition asks you to stop is what causes this pain. Your small intestine meridian is telling you that massage is no longer the right thing for you to do, but you ignore this and so block the energy flow in your small intestine meridian at point SI 11. See figure 8.7, page 265.

**What it feels like in your body:** An intense, often acute physical pain right in the center of the scapula.

## Pain at the Bottom Edge of the Scapula

Pain at the bottom edge of the scapula arises from giving yourself away or selling yourself short. In relationships, it is the pain of giving yourself to someone who doesn't love you or care about you. It can be the emotional pain of sadness from living a life that should not have turned out the way it did. Toward the end of life, it can be the pain of having to live the last years of your life on your own. The energy of this latter pain can run very deep and can work its way into the bone and become intense. On the spiritual level, the pain refers to your sacrificing your return "home," to the light, to infinite love and Spirit, in favor of a lifetime on Earth. To keep you attached to Earth, the ego grants you one big pay-off to keep you interested in life. This could be the joy and happiness of family, sex, emotional love, indulgence in pleasure, or success with money, power, intellect, or some attachment or pursuit that you are unwilling to break your attachment to. Although it may be a big thing to you in this lifetime, in comparison to a life of unlimited spirit and unconditional love, it is nothing. Thus your desire to stay here on Earth, especially toward the end of life, means you are selling yourself short. See figure 8.6, page 268.

**What it feels like in your body:** An intense, burning pain in the bone at the lowest edge of the scapula.

**Treatment for both pain in the center and bottom edge of the scapula:** As well as gentle massage of the scapula itself, additional care needs to be given to the front of the heart chakra. Heat needs to be generated in the heart chakra, through loving touch. The heat generated in the heart chakra can then flow into the small intestine meridian, which is linked to the fourth chakra, and this will help dissolve the blockage in the meridian along its running through the scapula. Be aware, however, that such relief is only temporary. The root of the pain is in lifestyle and the best thing a therapist can do is to impart this information as lovingly as possible to the client.

# 20. Upper-Arm Pain

In general, the upper arms, along with the elbows, forearms, wrists, and hands, are energetic extensions of the heart. Their condition is mirrored in the condition of the heart. If the heart is weak or closed, they will be weak or closed too. Similarly, the condition of the energy in the arms reflects back to the heart. Thus if there are blocks in energy in the arms, the heart becomes blocked too. For the heart to be free, the upper arms, elbows, forearms, wrists, and hands need to be free. Pain in the upper arms, elbows, forearms, wrists, and hands reveal a blockage in the energy flowing from the heart. They reveal that something about you or what you are doing in life is blocking your heart. This is the root of all arm pain. Arm pain indicates your heart is in pain.

Pain specifically in the upper arm indicates the pain of not opening your heart, or the accumulation of everything that has happened to you or that you have done in life that has blocked your heart from opening; for example, blaming others—usually your parents—for your own condition in life. By blaming your parents, you are not forgiving them. By not forgiving them, you are not loving them. By not loving them, you are blocking your heart from opening.

Upper-arm pain is often a complex, multilayered, intense pain, as the energy that is causing the discomfort runs through six meridians in the upper arm: the lung, large intestine, pericardium, triple heater, small intestine, and heart meridians. The types of subtle energy running through these meridians can be a mixture of emotional, mental, and behavioral energies, and accordingly manifest as different types of physical pain. Emotional energies running through these meridians are usually cold energies, such as loneliness, sadness about life, or the experience of having to live in a loveless marriage. These energies cause contraction, coldness, and heaviness in the muscles surrounding the running of these meridians. Other emotional energies, such as hatred for life or anger at a parent or spouse who has never loved you, cause hardness and tightness in the muscles. When the pain of life hurts you to the core of your very being, the accumulated energies can work themselves into the humerus bone itself and can be quite intense. Mental and behavioral energies running through the six meridians that block the heart from opening include the energies of unforgivingness, the need to inflict pain on someone who has hurt you, the need to build a wall of protection around yourself against an unloving parent or spouse, or blaming others for your own circumstances. These energies cause hardness and tightness in the muscles surrounding the running of these meridians. One specific behavioral energy, the one you use in holding on to your painful past, causes compression, pain, and weakness in the triceps, through which runs the large intestine meridian, the energetic function of which is to let go of the past. Compression in the triceps causes the arm to weaken when you try to raise it above your head.

Opening the heart, whether through yoga practice or therapeutic massage, will cause the six energy meridians in the upper arm to open. If a person opening their heart has experienced little or no love in life, the opening of the meridians will release great pain into your arm and will trigger the release of pain from other areas of the body, most noticeably from the latissimus and deltoid muscles, the rotator cuff, the bottom of the scapula, between the shoulder blades, the front of the fourth chakra, the back of the fourth chakra, the back of the third chakra, the area around L5 and S1, the tops of the hamstrings, the fronts of the thighs, the outsides of the thighs, and the dorsa of the feet. Yoga teachers and massage therapists experiencing such a complex energy release are often forced to rethink and reinvent their practice in order to protect themselves from this pain.

Not only do the six meridians in the upper arm store the energies of your own life that block the opening of your heart, they also house the energies of your parents. If your parents were unhappy together or if either or both of your parents experienced little or no love in their own lives, a second-generation copy of those cold energies is passed into you at the time of conception and houses itself in your upper arms. If you are at a stage of heart opening in your massage or yoga practice, you may find that you are not only releasing hurtful energies from your own past but also from the past of your parents.

There is no shortcut to opening your heart if there has been a lot of lovelessness in your life and in the lives of your parents. Emotionally, the heart will only open after the lung, large intestine, pericardium, triple heater, small intestine, and heart meridians have opened energetically. This process takes time, patience, understanding, and forgiveness. The heart meridian, as it opens, releases enormous heat and warmth running along the inside of the upper and lower arm, through the wrist, and out through the center of the palm of the hand. It is a wonderful energy. You can use it to bring great healing to others in your massage practice or to bring great physical strength to your arms in your yoga practice. See figure 8.8 and figure 8.9 on page 274.

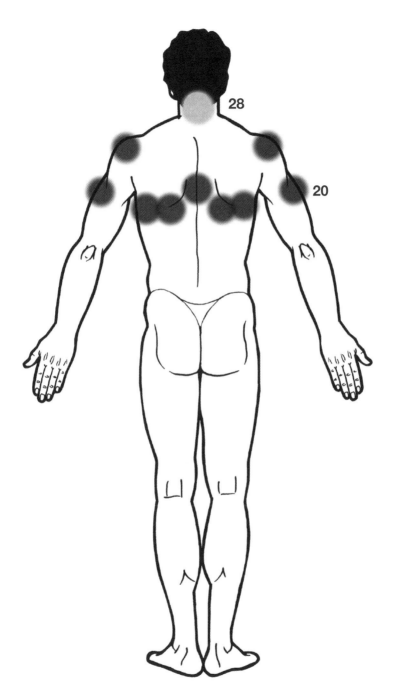

*Fig. 8.8. Pain on the back and side of the upper arm (20)
and tightness at the back of the neck (28)*

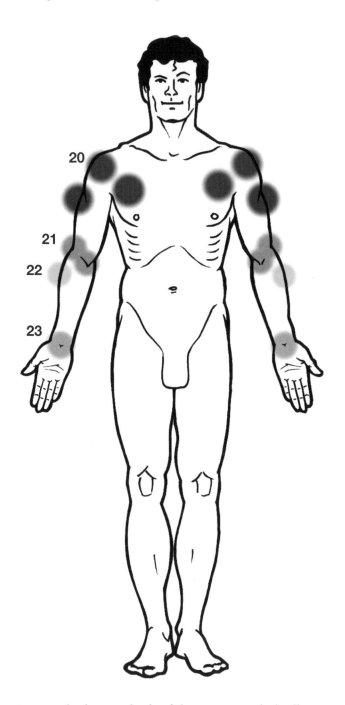

*Fig. 8.9. Pain on the front and side of the upper arm (20), elbow pain (21), tight forearm (22), and weak wrists (23)*

**What it feels like in your body:** Pain in this area is experienced as cold, compressed deltoids, or acute pain and weakness in the triceps.

**Treatment:** At the heart of upper-arm pain lies family history; for example, the pain of your parents having to live together although they did not love each other, the additional pain of one or both of your parents at not being loved by their own parents, and finally your own pain at being unloved—three generations of emotional pain that are linked together and that have become housed in your upper arm.

When seeking treatment for this pain, it can be useful to seek help from a professional who understands family dynamics and the patterns that run through and shape families. In addition, it can be beneficial to find a form of medical treatment that recognizes the role that energy, or chi, plays in the condition of the physical body, such as TCM acupuncture or shiatsu. Esoteric healers who recognize the role of energy in the body are also extremely useful to work with, including shamans, energy workers, or spiritual healers.

Self-development disciplines such as yoga or meditation can also be beneficial, but your teacher needs be experienced enough in their own self-development to be able to guide you through these painful releases. Massage too can be of help, but again, the therapist needs to be experienced enough to understand the possible underlying energetic origins of your physical pain. The treatment for upper arm pain in massage involves gentle massaging of the whole area between outer arm and heart, and warming the heart, the soft area above the heart, the outside of the rib cage, the armpit, and the shoulder. As well, establish a connection between the heart and the outer upper arm and enable the energy to flow from the heart into the whole upper arm.

## 21. Pain or Weakness inside the Elbow

Pain and weakness in the inside of the elbow is related to the pain of living your life through others—following others, being dependent on others, or seeking acceptance and validation from others. The behavior and need to seek validation from others blocks the path to your own freedom and to discovering your own authentic self. This block to freedom causes pain in your heart, the nature of which is to be free, and this is reflected in the elbows. See figure 8.9, page 274.

**What it feels like in your body:** The energy flow from your heart chakra is blocked in the running of the heart and pericardium meridians at the bottom edge of the humerus, causing pain to radiate from between the bottom of the humerus to the top of the ulna. An intense but dull pain, causing weakness in the elbow joint.

**Treatment:** In massage, cup the area in your hands and hold. Allow the heat of your hold to sink into the elbow joint. The joint itself does not require any form of physical manipulation. Additionally, massage the upper arm and front of the heart chakra and establish a connection between the energy of the heart and the elbow joint, running through the upper arm.

## 22. Forearm Tightness

Tightness in the forearm is related to the pain of being in service, of putting other people first, and the pain of putting other people's needs ahead of your own. This pain only arises when you have been trained to be in service by someone else, usually by a parent who has you so you can look after them. From your earliest days you were trained to live your life in accordance with the needs of others, your parents, and the only source of affirmation you received was in answering the needs of others. You grew up trained to feel happy in serving others. This is enslavement, and this is the message that you need to learn from this energy blockage. When, as an adult, you are completely free and happy to choose a life of service or not, this pain will not be present.

This is a common pain among massage therapists who find happiness and validation in their work. They find joy in their work because they have been trained by their parents to find happiness in serving the needs of others. If they were truly and completely free in their work and working from this place of complete freedom, from where the energy of their heart could flow freely through their arms, then there would be no blockages in their forearms. The blockage in the forearm reveals they are not free in their massage work, although they believe they are. It is a very contentious issue! See figure 8.9, page 274.

**What it feels like in your body:** Tightness or mild hardness in the extensor carpi ulnaris and digitorum muscles.

**Treatment:** Gentle, loving massage of the posterior forearm. This can also be done with self-massage.

## 23. Weak Wrists

Weakness in the wrists is related to the belief that you need to belong to a group, as without group affirmation or support you believe you are in a position of weakness. It involves a belief in weakness—that you are too weak to stand on your own two feet. If you believe you are weak, the weakness will be reflected physically in your body. Similar to the condition of weakness in the elbow joint, the pain resides in the heart and pericardium meridians, this time at the bottom of the ulna. See figure 8.9, page 274.

**What it feels like in your body:** Weakness in the muscular strength in the wrist.

**Treatment:** Cup the wrist in your hands and hold. Allow the heat of your hold to sink into the wrist joint. The joint does not require any form of physical manipulation, although there is no harm in giving it some gentle manipulation. With your hold, generate a feeling of love and loving intention in your touch and work to move this energy into the wrist of the client. The energy of love is what is needed to heal the weakness.

## 24. Pain in the Right Arm

There is a specific type of subtle energy that causes pain in your right arm and in your heart: the energy of another person's jealousy of you.

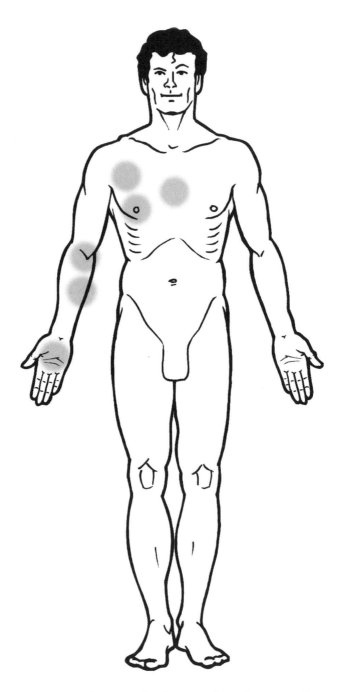

*Fig. 8.10. The pain of jealousy in the right arm and in
the right-hand side of the fourth chakra (24)*

Jealousy is a hurtful energy, and another person's jealousy of you can cause you hurt, especially to your heart and your right arm. When you come into physical contact with someone who is jealous of you, the energy of their jealousy enters your energetic body through the palm of your right hand and travels up your right arm along the pericardium meridian toward your heart. Your pericardium will then intuitively work to block the flow of this incoming energy, causing a blockage and resulting in the physical manifestation of a painful inflammation in your lower arm. The right side of the body is the side through which you draw in energy to yourself, while the left side is the side through which you release and let go of energy. The energy of another person's jealousy of you can also enter your body through the center of your right nipple. This leads to blockage, resistance, and stiffness in the body area above the right nipple, including your right shoulder and upper right arm. It can also cause a rise in blood pressure. See figure 8.10.

**What it feels like in the body of a massage client:** A feeling of coldness and slight heaviness in the lower arm or in the soft tissue between heart and clavicle.

**Treatment:** Massage treatment involves metaphysically pulling all the energy of jealousy out of the body of the client, either through their right hand or through their right nipple, until none of it is left. This is specialized, hands-off energetic work, usually carried out by an appropriately trained shaman, energy worker, or spiritual healer.

## 25. Coldness between the Upper Chest and the Clavicle

The energies of current or former loneliness (black in color), grief (gray), sadness (yellow), or despair (dark green) are housed in the area of the body between the upper chest and the clavicle. See figure 8.11, page 280.

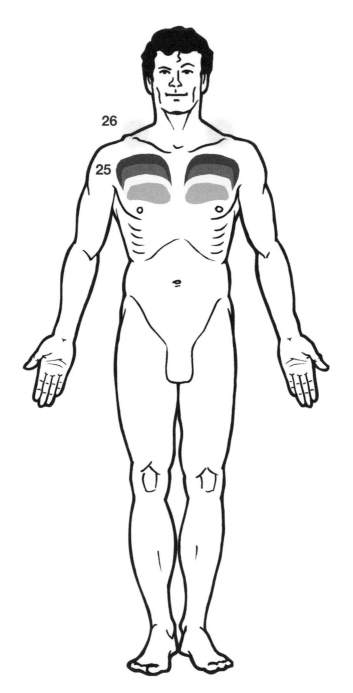

*Fig. 8.11. Coldness between the upper chest and clavicle (25)
and pain in the trapezius (26)*

**What it feels like in the body of a massage client:** The area feels soft and spongy to the touch, and cold when you hold your hand above it. In your own body the energies of grief and sadness metaphysically manifest as a fog or mist that sits between you and your direct experience of your environment. The resulting feeling is one of a loss of connection to life.

**Treatment:** Place you hand on the sternum and use the natural warmth and weight of your hand to soften the area. The heat from your hand will also enable your client to breathe more into the area, which will help release the energies held here. You can aid the release by gently massaging the area. Work with great sensitivity. In some instances your client may weep or cry during treatment.

## 26. Pain in the Trapezius

This is TCM gallbladder point GB 21, on the top of the shoulder directly above the nipple, known as the shoulder well, and no wonder. It is the point on the gallbladder meridian that carries the energy of our belief in our own limitations. It also fires the energy of frustration arising from such a belief. This point can become sensitive and very painful when massaged during times when we feel frustrated by our personal limitations, such as not having the confidence to ask our boss for a pay raise. The more we focus on such limitation, the stronger and more painful the energy in this gallbladder point becomes. See figure 8.11.

**What it feels like in your body:** Physical tightness in the trapezius muscle. This can be an incredibly painful point on the top of the shoulder.

**Treatment:** Gentle, not vigorous, massage treatment of the trapezius supported with additional heart chakra work, opening and warming the chakra and imparting reassurance, strength, and love through the energetic quality of your touch to your client.

# 27. Inflammation
# at the Sides of the Neck

Inflammation or swelling at the sides of the neck is caused by a blockage in the energy needed to speak freely. When it is found in a location from the back of the neck to the sides of the neck, it involves the self-control you exert against speaking your feelings or needs, against speaking your truth. You may do this out of fear of being judged, out of fear of being rejected by your audience, or out of fear of having some form of personal power taken away from you, as by the comment "What a stupid thing to say," which undermines your intelligence. When the condition is found in the area from the front of the neck to the sides of the neck it relates to the direct control or pressure a specific person puts on you against speaking your true feelings or needs; for example, the pressure an employer puts on you to not criticize their unfair treatment of you, or the pressure a controlling parent puts on you not to criticize them. When the block to speaking freely is severe, it travels upward into the lower jaw, where it tightens and contracts the jaw muscles. See figure 8.12.

**What it feels like in your body and in the body of a massage client:** Soft, cool, spongy inflammation in the sides of the neck. The cool energy, indicating the emotional energy of fear, additionally causes weakness in the muscles in the neck.

**Treatment:** Suggest that your massage client find a free space out in nature or by the sea, where they can vent their feelings. The energy of blocked communication needs to be released. Do not suggest venting their feelings in the car, as the energy of their anger will just bounce off the windshield and back into their neck and throat. Similarly, do not suggest direct confrontation.

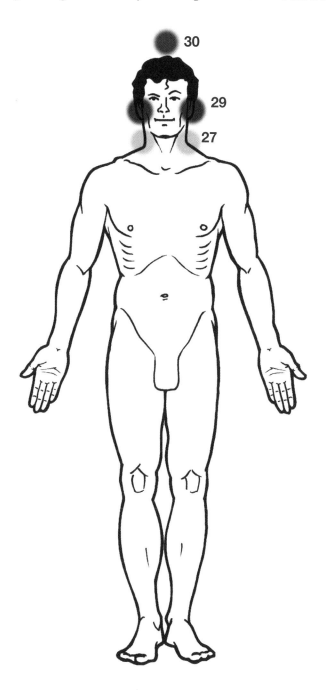

*Fig. 8.12. Inflammation at the sides of the neck (27), ear pain (29),
and the location of crown energy (30)*

## 28. Tightness at the Back of the Neck

The point of indecision: when you can't decide what to do when you know you have to make a decision about your future and all the options have been put before you. Can't see the future. Can't see what's coming. See figure 8.8, on page 273.

> **What it feels like in your body:** A pinching in the area just below the atlas between C3 and C5
>
> **Treatment:** Massage the area gently until warm and soft. Support with additional work on the sixth and seventh chakras, the shoulder blades, and the heart, energetically connecting all four body areas together.

## 29. Ear, Head, and Neck Pain

The ears are the portals through which the energy of words spoken to us enters our system. Words of love, truth, good advice, and support naturally carry good energy with them, and when this energy enters our body it creates warmth and openness wherever it goes. Words of hatred, violence, deceit, manipulation, or control carry damaging energy with them, and when these words enter our body through our ears, their energy causes the ears and the areas around the ears to tighten and harden in an act of protection and defense. Such words can also result in headache and tightness in the neck. The reason for this happening is that as the damaging energy of hurtful words travels downward throughout the body from the ears, it tries to pass through the fourth chakra, the area of the heart. The heart, however, is able to discern truth from untruth, and what is good for us and what is not good for us, and so it blocks the downward flow of harmful word energy, causing blockage of energy in the head and neck. I have seen this kind of energy block manifest in yoga teachers who go to the workshops of highly regarded teachers, yet come away with a blinding headache and a vaguely intuitive feeling that the yoga teacher does not fully understand what it is they are teaching. The heart of the student, which already knows that the teacher does not know what they are talking about, blocks the energy of the words of the teacher, causing energy blockages in the areas above the heart: the throat, neck, and head. This is a sign that the student has outgrown the teacher and now needs to move on from that person. The same thing happens when someone with an open heart goes to listen to the words of a spiritual guru who uses words of wisdom with the hidden intention of needing to control his audience or the need to build a discipleship. Such an openhearted person will leave the experience with a blinding headache. See figure 8.12, page 283.

**What it feels like in the body of a massage client:** The cartilage of the ear feels thicker than usual and there is resistance to bending or folding it. There is also a thin layer of dense, semi-hardness in front of the ear, behind the ear, and above the ear. The portion of neck below the ear is similarly semihard and is cold to the touch.

**Treatment:** Gentle, slow massage of the whole area. It is better to cup the back of the neck in your hand and squeeze it gently instead of massaging it. Hold the squeeze grip and as you feel the neck soften, slowly and gently increase the pressure of the squeeze until the neck is completely soft. Use finger pressure around the ear. Slow, warm, circular movements. Start gently, but gradually increase pressure as the tissue softens and the layer of denseness goes. Rub your hands together until hot and place over the ears. Repeat until the ears turn red or become warm.

## 30. The Crown

For some students of yoga, the spiritual aspects of yoga, ruled by the sixth and seventh chakras, or ajna and crown chakras, become an important element of their practice. Seeking guidance in this area to help them further deepen their practice, they are drawn to workshops offered by well-established, often globally recognized teachers of their chosen system of yoga. Students assume a world-renowned teacher of yoga understands all aspects of yoga, including a full understanding of the more abstract, symbolic, spiritual aspects. The trouble is, some world-renowed yoga teachers in the West do not understand the deeper, more hidden spiritual wisdoms of yoga, which is a tradition of the East. They therefore misinterpret some of the spiritual teachings and then share these misinterpretations with their students. The students, in innocence, openly accept these misinterpretations. Because of the nature of the subject matter involved, spirituality, the energy of misinterpreted spiritual wisdom causes blockages in the spiritual centers: the sixth and seventh chakras.

The color of energy at the center of the seventh chakra is very bright white. The color of the energy of misunderstanding and misinterpretation is black. Misinterpreted teachings on the spiritual aspects of yoga show up as blobs of black energy in the center of the seventh chakra. There are no physical side effects; however, they do block the energy of true spiritual understanding from subsequently entering the energy system of the yoga student. See figure 8.12, page 283.

**What it feels like in the body of a massage client:** Place your hand flat above the crown of the client. This area normally feels warm. If cold, it reveals a blockage. If you are a therapist sensitive to the colors of energy, you will sense the color black over the crown.

**Treatment:** Seek help from an appropriately trained shaman, energy worker, or spiritual healer. Ask them to check the condition of the energy in your seventh chakra. Treatment of the condition involves the removal of the blocking energy from the crown. Some healers may achieve this by drumming the energy out of your crown, others by sending it to the light, while others will simply swish it away with their hands.

# Becoming the Person You Were Meant to Be

Stress is a subconscious conflict caused by the distance between the person you were born to be and the person you have become. The more life has led you away from your true self, the person you were born to be, the greater the level of stress you will experience. Stress is a way of letting you know you are going in the wrong direction. Stress can therefore be an opportunity to pause and take stock, and, if necessary, to alter the direction of your life to better align with your true direction.

If you are serious about wanting a less stressful life, one of the most important things you can do is discover your authentic self, the person you were born to be, the life you were meant to live, your destiny. This can be achieved by working with a shaman, energy worker, clairvoyant, astrologer, or spiritualist and asking them if they can help you discover your soul's purpose and the life tasks you have chosen for yourself. You are the only person who knows what you have set yourself to accomplish in this lifetime. It is set within you, and when you do not follow your true path, the result is inner conflict. The person you were born to be is your true destiny. It is the life path your spirit freely chose for you before you were conceived and is an expression of your free will. Difficulty arises because by the time you have gathered all the skills necessary to enact the life you have chosen for yourself, through years of education, etc., you have forgotten the type of life you originally chose for yourself. Having forgotten the life you chose for yourself, you followed a lifestyle that others or society chose for you. This is the root cause of conflict in life, the kind of conflict that causes stress.

Let's say, for example, that before you were born into the world you chose the life of a teacher, a spiritual teacher. You accept that in order to fulfill this role you will have to make some sort of connection to spiritual energy during your lifetime here. You know you will need good communication skills. You also realize that you may have to stand on your own two feet, as what you intend to teach may go against the opinions and understandings of others. To help you fulfill your destiny, you will need a personality type that is suited to expressing ideas and communicating. You also need a personality type that is strongly independent, so you can be someone who can stand on your own two feet.

Throughout history the idea of personality type or archetype has been well-documented, with the most common personality types that repeat throughout history well described. Some archetypes are described psychoanalytically, such as those described by Jung, while others are described esoterically, such as those described in certain systems of astrology or in the tarot. Knowing the personality type or archetype and the characteristics you will need to help you more easily achieve your destiny on Earth is important. Before you incarnate you choose those personality characteristics from the classifications of personality types or archetypes that have already been described. So, in this example of the person with the destiny to be a spiritual teacher, knowing you will need communication skills, you choose a personality classification that reflects communication, a personality type described as Gemini in Western astrology. You also choose a classification that reflects independence and contentment in independence, a personality type described as Tiger in the Chinese zodiac system. You then work out when in time, Gemini and Tiger cross, and this determines your birth date. The astrological signs of Gemini and Tiger are two clues you leave for yourself to help you understand the destiny you have chosen for yourself and the type of life and lifestyle you have chosen for yourself. Your given name is also a classification of personality type. Names have meaning. The name you are given by your parents is often the name you have chosen for yourself. Research the meaning of your name and understand that it too is a clue to your destiny.

So to continue with the example that you have chosen for yourself, the life of a spiritual teacher, to help fulfill this destiny you will need to make some sort of connection to spiritual energy in your life, as through this connection the necessary spiritual wisdom will follow. In our modern, urban, employment-focused Western world, connection to spiritual wisdom during the formative years is neither well-received nor strongly encouraged. As a child grows up and goes through the educational system, encouragement is given for other aspects of life, such as sports, artistic creativity, language and writing skills, math, science, and the development of other specific skills necessary for employment or for higher education. There is no room for spiritual development, such as training in animism, shamanism, or meditation. So the child, having chosen for herself the role of spiritual teacher, is faced with life choices that do not fit her destiny. This is why it is not uncommon to find that certain lifestyles and careers simply do not work for you. They do not work for you because none of them are the ones you have already chosen for yourself, your true calling in life. Sometimes you have to wait until your late twenties, thirties, or early forties before you can find your true path in life, your thirties being the period of life during which the centers of spiritual energy, the fifth and sixth chakras, naturally open.

So how do you reduce the level of life stress you are currently enduring and discover your true destiny? Look for the clues you have left for yourself. Explore astrology and fields of spiritual development. Seek guidance from people trained to be life guides: astrologers, clairvoyants, mediums, channelers, shamans. Pray. Pray to someone you feel you can trust. This may be a historical or even a living figure. Ask for guidance. It is not unusual to have someone in your current lifetime who knows you well and whom you can trust, who also happens to be one of your spirit guides, a member of your karmic or spirit family. This is often a grandparent or someone from the generation before your parents. If you have no one like this in your life, then choose a historical figure for guidance. Aim high, go to the top, to exceptional guides and teachers: Buddha, Abraham, Mohammed, Jesus. If you do not like the idea of communicating with a historical figure associated with a religion, just remember that none of them were considered religious figures when they were alive. They were simply human beings who were later turned into religious figures. Whomever you choose, make direct contact with your chosen figure. Don't bother with intermediaries. When you connect with them, ask them for help in discovering your true nature. Maybe the answer will come to you in a dream, or maybe somebody will be sent to you who will help you find the answer.

When you begin to uncover the life you first chose for yourself and then begin to make changes in your life that will bring you into closer alignment with that choice, you will find your levels of life stress dramatically fall away, and you will also find greater happiness.

## A Simple Test to See How Free You Are

This is a fun and easy test I learned from my energy teacher in Chiang Mai, Jasmine Vishnu, while studying with her in the early 2000s. To do this test you need to be at peace in mind and in body. You can do it during savasana in yoga, or lying in bed before you go to sleep, or by just sitting down in a chair in your living room when you have a period of uninterrupted free time.

- Start by visualizing something that is easy and neutral, such as an inanimate object, something you have no connection with, say, a street sign or a lamppost. Most people have no emotional connection with lampposts, so imagine a lamppost in front of you. Using your imagination, draw the lamppost toward you, and then pass it through and behind you. You should have no difficulty with this.

- Try the exercise again, this time visualize a person, someone you have no connection to, maybe someone you saw in a newspaper or in a school history book. Make it a person with whom you have no emotional involvement, so no movie or sports stars you admire, just a John or Jane Doe. Imagine them standing in front of you. In your imagination draw them toward you and then allow them to pass through you. If they pass right through you, there is no connection between you and that person. They are free of you. You are free of them.

- Now repeat this exercise with someone you know, say, a friend, a colleague, or someone from your yoga class. Bring the person into your imagination and beckon them to walk through you. Do they pass right through you, or as they pass through you does some part of their body get stuck in yours? Do they leave behind something in you as they walk through you? The getting-stuck experience is perfectly reproduced in the movie *Terminator 2,* where Robert Patrick's liquid metal T-1000 tries to walk through the prison bars at the state hospital where Sarah Connors is being held, but gets stuck three quarters through by his solid metal gun. In this example, you are the prison bars. If the person gets stuck in you as they try to walk through you, it shows that there is something not clear in your relationship with that person. There is a hidden sticking point in your friendship or relationship. The area in your body where the person gets stuck as they pass through you helps reveal the nature of what it is that is not clear between the two of you. For instance, if someone walking through you gets stuck in the region of your upper chest, it may indicate that the person is jealous of you in some way. Maybe in your yoga class there is a fellow student who is secretly jealous of you, your practice, or your physique. Conversely, it may also indicate that you are somehow jealous of another person. If you do this exercise with a friend with whom there is unfinished financial business, they will get stuck in your solar plexus as they try to walk through you. Doing this exercise reveals how free you are with the friends in your life.
- Once you have successfully gone through all your friends, start on your lovers, all of them. Check to see if they can all walk through you. Discover which of your exes still has unfinished business with you.
- Finally, do this exercise with the most important people of all, your family—mother, father, sister, brother. See if they can walk through you. If they get stuck on the way through, it shows there are unresolved issues between you and that family member.

If in doing the exercise you find a person you cannot even draw close to you, it reveals you are completely blocked with that person. Maybe this was a parent who was cruel to you for many years. This shows there is no degree of freedom between you and that person. When you have tried this exercise using all your friends, lovers, and family members, and they have all freely passed through you, then you are indeed free. As long as there is someone who cannot walk through you, you are not free.

This is a particularly telling exercise for people who believe that freedom comes with the pursuit of pleasure or from the accumulation and spending of wealth.

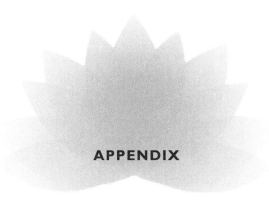

# The Esoteric

This is a small section offering insights into certain dreams and symbols that by their nature do not easily fall into the eight categories of subtle energy detailed throughout the book. Their inclusion here is merely as a means of aiding a better understanding of these phenomena, especially if you have experienced them yourself.

## "Past Life" Dreams

Past lives don't tend to come up and meet you on the street; they tend to visit you in your dreams. Sometimes these dreams are very vivid and contain a great many details. This makes them feel real and makes what they portray feel somehow real too, like they are describing an actual past-life experience. They tend to portray you in a series of life circumstances you logically know are not part of your current life. In an attempt to rationalize this type of portrayal, you call it a dream of a past life. It is, however, a dream, and the way a dream of such a so-called past life communicates with you is the same way any other dream does: through symbols.

Some symbols in these kinds of dreams are flattering and pleasant, such as being a goddess or a knight in shining armor. We tend not to question these dreams, accepting them on face value. Some of these "past life" dream symbols, however, can be deeply disturbing, such as a dream in which you are being tortured. In the dream, you may even feel the acute pain of the torture. You see the room in which you are being tortured, you see the uniforms your torturers are wearing, you see them torturing you, you even see their instruments of torture. The vividness and detail of the dream leads you to reason it must have really happened in some past life. But did it? Or is the dream a symbolic retelling of another story. And if so, what?

The next time you begin to experience an uncomfortable dream of what seems to be a past life, wake yourself up into a state of semiwakefulness, but deep enough to allow the dream to remain. Consciously ask that the dream be replayed to you in a way you can better understand it. Allow yourself to fall back to sleep again and see what happens. Most likely you will be given a very quick glimpse of a painful event that happened in your present life. This event may have been so painful that it is very hard for you to confront it head-on, so your mind sends you the event in the form of a dream that you can face, although it is still very uncomfortable. The purpose of such a "past life" dream is to get you to release negative mental energy you are still holding in your body that relates to that painful event that occurred in your present lifetime. It is a part of the process of letting go. That is what such a "past life" dream experience is: a retelling of a part of your current life in a way that is easier for you to deal with.

Some of these kinds of dreams are not so vivid. They seem to be exactly the opposite, in fact. Darker, without much light, not much environmental detail, and less emotional content. Everything feels hundreds and hundreds of years old. These kinds of dreams feel like really old past lives, maybe your first lifetime on Earth. A common symbol of a "first life on Earth" dream is a burning house, a house you have run out of. The more historical the past life feels, the closer it is to being a retelling of something from your earliest childhood. But again, what seemingly feels like a past-life experience of your first lifetime on Earth is merely a symbolic retelling of your first experiences in your current lifetime. In fact, the "past life" dreams with the least amount of detail are often a retelling of events that happened while you were still in the womb. The reason why there are so few details in these early-life dreams is that when you were in your earliest childhood your senses were not yet sufficiently developed to build a fully sense-based interpretation of your environment. At that age you were capable of registering only parts of your environment, which later in adulthood are reproduced in terms of specific past life dream experiences.

You may disagree with this insight—many will—but the way to find out is to wake yourself up in your next so-called past life dream and ask for the dream to be replayed to you in a way you can more easily interpret and understand. More than likely an image from early childhood from your present life will arise.

## Being Suffocated by a Big Black Blob

I know I am not the only one to have had the big black blob experience. The dream of being held down and suffocated by a big black blob is very frightening. You wake up completely paralyzed, unable to breathe. There is an intensely deep black figure on top of you, holding you down. It takes enormous effort to set yourself free of this dream.

If you have had this frightening experience and want to know what it means, the first thing you need to reflect on is whether the black blob was at all times in direct contact with you. In other words, it did not travel from across your bedroom to your bed and jump on you from there; when you woke up it was already on you, it already had a connection with you. In this experience, the black presence is a projection of blackness from within yourself. The blackness is the energy of fear, deep fear. This is the energy of a very deep fear you once experienced and is an experience that would almost suffocate you if you were to relive it. The suffocating black blob is your body releasing the energy of deep fear from within you. As the energy leaves your body from your subconscious, it passes through the layer of your consciousness, bringing the hidden experience temporarily back into your awareness, causing you to wake up. Although this is a very frightening experience, it is an incredibly positive one, as it shows your body slowly healing itself of a previously extremely fearful event by slowly letting its energy go.

It is not uncommon for the black blob to revisit you, but the good news is that each time it does, its power diminishes. Its color will change, too, from black to dark gray, to light gray, to grayish white, and finally to white. You will find yourself increasingly able to breathe, to move, and even to talk during each subsequent dream experience. By the end of this process you will be completely comfortable and able to easily talk to the blob. The letting go happens incrementally over time, not all at once. As you let go bit by bit, you become increasingly less frightened of the blob.

## Dreams of Being Strangled

A dream of being strangled is a joyous sign of spiritual awakening, as noted in the discussion of spiritual energy in chapter 5. The two things to note in a dream of this kind are that you are being strangled, or held tightly, around your neck, the location of the fifth chakra, the chakra that houses the energy of truth; and that you are being strangled by a male figure or character. The male figure is a symbol of the ego, the third chakra, the chakra that houses the energy of reason and rational, logical thought. What the dream signifies is the threat posed to your rational, conscious mind by the awakening of your higher centers of energy, which will, in turn, awaken the corresponding higher levels of spiritual consciousness and understanding. The conscious mind, as symbolized by the male figure in the dream, is threatened by the awakening of the higher energy centers and tries to block the energy of the higher chakras from moving downward through your body into your heart chakra. It does this by symbolically trying to strangle the flow of downward-moving energy at your neck.

Don't worry if you have a dream like this. You are in no danger. Neither is anyone else. No one is going to be strangled. No one is going to die. The only thing that will happen is that your thinking about life will change, and most likely for the better.

The heart and, by extension, the heart chakra is the seat of full understanding. Spiritual insight about life is able to enter your seat of full understanding without the need for reasoning or rational explanations. This is done by opening and growing the energy in your higher-energy centers, the fifth and sixth chakras, and then moving this energy downward into your heart chakra, where it triggers the wonderful lightbulb moment of insight and deep understanding.

Let's say you are going to listen to a lecture from a spiritual teacher. In such a situation you are usually seated in a hall or lecture room. During the lecture the spiritual energy in the words of the teacher will open and fill your sixth chakra. As it does, lightly bring your awareness and your breath to your sixth chakra and, as you exhale, move your awareness downward from your sixth into your fourth chakra, bringing the energy of the teacher's words with it.

Integrating spiritual wisdom poses a threat to the energy of your rational mind, as a spiritual understanding of life challenges one's logical, conscious understanding of life, often revealing the rational understanding of life to in fact be a *misunderstanding* of life. Your conscious mind, not wanting to be revealed as not being right, tries to block the truthfulness that results from your spiritual awakening!

## The Alchemist

The Alchemist is an archetypal figure found throughout history. The role of the Alchemist, that of turning base metal into gold, is often taken too literally and too seriously, however; there is no chemistry or science involved in this universal archetype.

The beauty of the Alchemist archetype is that anybody can be the alchemist. You don't even have to know anything about metal! The true meaning of the Alchemist archetype is that it represents the person who is capable of turning commonly accepted beliefs about life on their heads, to reveal the hidden spiritual truth about them.

Base metal is a double symbol. A base represents a root, a foundation. The base chakra is the root chakra, the first chakra. Metal is a symbol used to describe the energy form that gives rise to the structures of human conscious belief. This is a completely different symbol than the symbol of metal used in Five Elements theory in TCM, or the element of metal attributed to the lungs. Base metal in the Alchemist archetype represents the store of collective human consciousness, which has been passed to us through our ancestors and through our own past lives and which is found in the first chakra.

Gold is the color used to describe energy of a very high vibration, commonly attributed to the seventh chakra and higher. It is an energy that represents the wealth and abundance that comes to you following the completion of your life tasks and the gaining of a full understanding of your life (this is discussed in more detail in chapter 2, pages 78–79, "Balancing All the Chakras"). Energy of a gold color can be found in various forms of meditation and other spiritual practices. It is usually found outside the body, above the seventh chakra, where it can be drawn into the body through the crown and downward along the spinal column.

The energy of understanding that lies at the first or root chakra, base metal, is born without full understanding. Hence the journey of the Alchemist is to bring the energy of full understanding, gold, to the energy of the human conscious understanding that you are born with, base metal. This journey may also be described as being the journey toward enlightenment. The archetype of the Alchemist is also attributed to the person whose life starts in unpeaceful circumstances but ends in peace.

## "I Am a Ray of Light"

Some gurus and healers like to say they are special "rays of light" sent to Earth from distant galaxies to help heal everyone here on Earth. This is very nice. Well, there is even nicer news: everyone on this planet is a ray of light. Everyone, without exception.

Just as "past life" dreams are in reality a symbolic retelling of an event from your current life, the dream or meditative vision of being a ray of light is a symbolic way for you to see yourself without your physical form. It is just you, the person you truly are, seen in a different form, in a different light, as it were. If you ever do see yourself as a ray of light, either in a dream, a meditation, or in other spiritual practices, it means you are in a temporary state of raised consciousness, higher than your normal consciousness that places you in this three-dimensional world. The ability to see yourself as a ray of light reveals that your higher chakras, five, six, and seven, are open, allowing you to see yourself from a different dimension.

Rays of light are of pure white light. The white light, however, can become refracted as it passes through the earth to reveal different colors of the spectrum, from red to violet, in the same way light is refracted by rain to reveal a rainbow. This is why some gurus claiming to be rays of light say they are of different colors of light, or rainbow-hued. The different refracted colors of the ray of white light also mark the seven different chakras in our body.

Deep, dark purple is one of the refracted colors. Deep, dark purple is also the color of one of the energies that happens to pass through Earth on its journey through the cosmos from one unknown place toward another unknown place. This is why some people who dream or envision being a ray of light with a deep, dark purple color interpret this as meaning they are a ray of light that has come from a distant part of the galaxy. There is no harm in a guru claiming to be a ray of light from a distant galaxy sent to Earth to do good. Tell them you are, too!

Any person who claims to be a ray of light yet doesn't recognize that everyone they meet is also a ray of light reveals that they are not what they say they are. In the realm of light, all is light. It cannot be that one person is light while another is not. There is no duality. There is no "I am a ray of light and you are not."

In dreams and meditations, the symbol of the ray of light is also one that can be used to traverse the space that lies between the separated internal male and female energies within the body.

# Index

Page numbers in *italic* refer to illustrations.

# Books of Related Interest

**The Subtle Energy Body**
The Complete Guide
*by Maureen Lockhart, Ph.D.*

**Vibrational Medicine**
The #1 Handbook of Subtle-Energy Therapies
*by Richard Gerber, M.D.*

**Tuning the Human Biofield**
Healing with Vibrational Sound Therapy
*by Eileen Day McKusick*

**The Healing Intelligence of Essential Oils**
The Science of Advanced Aromatherapy
*by Kurt Schnaubelt, Ph.D.*

**Chakras**
Energy Centers of Transformation
*by Harish Johari*

**Crystal and Stone Massage**
Energy Healing for the Vital and Subtle Bodies
*by Michael Gienger*

**Hot Stone and Gem Massage**
*by Dagmar Fleck and Liane Jochum*

**Microchakras**
InnerTuning for Psychological Well-being
*by Sri Shyamji Bhatnagar and David Isaacs, Ph.D.*

INNER TRADITIONS • BEAR & COMPANY
P.O. Box 388
Rochester, VT 05767
1-800-246-8648
www.InnerTraditions.com

Or contact your local bookseller